The author is a Korean war navy veteran. He is a graduate of Duquesne University and is retired after working forty years in manufacturing operations management. He is a native of Pittsburgh who now resides in Ft. Myers, Florida.

John Siko

ANATOMY OF A WRONGFUL DEATH LAWSUIT

AUSTIN MACAULEY PUBLISHERS™

LONDON * CAMBRIDGE * NEW YORK * SHARJAH

Copyright © John Siko 2024

All rights reserved. No part of this publication may be reproduced, distributed, or transmitted in any form or by any means, including photocopying, recording, or other electronic or mechanical methods, without the prior written permission of the publisher, except in the case of brief quotations embodied in critical reviews and specific other non-commercial uses permitted by copyright law. For permission requests, write to the publisher.

Any person who commits any unauthorized act about this publication may be liable to criminal prosecution and civil claims for damages.

The story, experiences, and words are the author's alone.

Ordering Information
Quantity sales: Special discounts are available on quantity purchases by corporations, associations, and others. For details, contact the publisher at the address below.

Publisher's Cataloging-in-Publication data
Siko, John
Anatomy of a Wrongful Death Lawsuit

ISBN 9798889102991 (Paperback)
ISBN 9798889103004 (ePub e-book)

Library of Congress Control Number: 2024900082

www.austinmacauley.com/us

First Published 2024
Austin Macauley Publishers LLC
40 Wall Street, 33rd Floor, Suite 3302
New York, NY 10005
USA

mail-usa@austinmacauley.com
+1 (646) 5125767

Table of Contents

Chapter 1
The Beginning

I didn't know that 12 May 2017 would be the beginning of my life's most extended four years.

Returning home from running an errand, I found my wife, Beth, on the floor with Coke spread all over the wall and floor. She informed me that she had slipped and fallen earlier and could not get up. I tried lifting her onto a chair, but she was deadweight and complained about how much her knee hurt.

She was hurt far worse than first suspected, and my attempt to get her on the chair might worsen the injury. I decided she needed to go to the emergency room (ER) and made a 911 call to have her transported by ambulance. EMS arrived, stabilized her, and agreed with my decision to move her to the ER, telling me it would take about an hour to get her admitted.

After waiting an hour, I drove to the emergency room and learned she was going through the admitting process and that the nurse would call me when I could visit her.

Let me digress here and detail an emergency room in a Florida hospital. As you enter the waiting room, it will feel like you have just entered a meat cooler; it is cold. You will see a room full of potential patients; some in wheelchairs; some lying across two or three seats trying to sleep; some—if they could get one—wrapped in a blanket to keep warm; others with their noses in their iPhones. If you are not wearing a sweater, you would be better off waiting in the parking lot where it is warm.

Upon entering, you go to the admitting desk, where the first information they ask is whether you have insurance. If you pass that test, they ask why you are there. Your case goes in a gray folder; you are given a wristband with your name and sent back into the waiting room. People who have used the ER before are wise enough to say they have chest pains whether they do or not. They get a red folder and move immediately to get an EKG; they may find something wrong with your heart.

In most cases, the EKG shows nothing, and you lose your red folder and are put into a gray one and returned to the waiting room to join the first-come, first-served patients. Depending on the month of the year, you may or may not get a seat in the waiting room. Southwest Florida is in the migratory path of the snowbirds, and many roost here. Having no local doctor, they use the ER as their fallback option to treat their headaches, stomach aches, or just because they do not feel well but do not know why.

The local saying is, "Do not get sick between November and April and go to the ER because you may face a two—to three-hour wait to be seen." If you are making a trip to the ER, bring a book. However, you may be able to find reading material left in the waiting area by patients that have moved to the business area of the emergency room. The available literature may include the *Christine Science Monitor,* the *Enquire*, and other dog-eared magazines.

When called, you go from a freezing waiting room to an icy ER area. Depending on your condition, you may get a room, a gurney in the hallway, or a reclining chair. If you get a room, they take off your clothes and put you in a private gown—a male or female nurse wearing a floral blouse, checkered pants, and sneakers will visit. You do not know if they are there to take your blood or take out the trash. It is pretty different from when Beth was a nurse. It was a clean white dress, polished shoes, a cap you spent hours starching and ironing, and your nurse's pin.

Even though the nursing attire has changed, it has not affected their professionalism, and Beth never complained about the care she received from all the nurses that treated her. They were professional and caring despite their attire. If you get a gurney, you have a curtain pulled around the bed, changing in the hall. You get a chair if you have a symptom that does not require lying down. Now the wait begins once again for a doctor to see you. When they show up, they ask what brought you here today and instruct the nurse to draw blood.

Usually, the blood work results determine your problem and whether it is severe enough to admit you. The wait time for a doctor to see you is 30 to 40 minutes, and blood work results take three to four hours. Remember, no one in the waiting room can be admitted to the emergency room until one of the room, gurney, or chair patients leave.

Beth, brought by ambulance, expedited the check-in process, and the nurse placed her on a gurney in the hall. After a review by the doctor, he sent her for an x-ray for pictures of her leg. Once again, the waiting begins in the cold ER hallway, but Beth is lucky enough to get a blanket.

An hour later, the doctor said, "The good news is there are no fractures," and told the nurse to give my wife a 'road test.' If she passed, she could go home. The medical definition of a 'road test' is: "To assess discharge suitability criteria by the testing level of self-sufficiency, cerebellar function-gait, ataxia, ambulation and the ability to understand discharge instructions."

The medical definition of ambulation states, "The ability to walk from place to place independently with or without assistive devices."

The ER nurse got a walker and asked Beth to stand. With the assistance of the walker and much difficulty, she managed to stand but complained about how much her leg hurt, telling the nurse she was having tremendous pain in her left knee and could not take a step without the pain increasing. I asked the nurse to see if she could walk to the bathroom without pain, but she said she had passed the 'road test' by standing up and weight-bearing on the injured leg with an assist from the walker.

She informed me there were no fractures; pain usually follows a fall. I told the Case Worker, who works with the discharge nurse, and explained the discharge procedure; Beth needs to remain in the hospital on an observation basis. She said this was expensive since Medicare would not pay for this type of admittance unless a diagnosis showed the patient had a medical necessity. I said I would be willing to pay the fee because I believed further examination would show she had an undiagnosed problem that further investigation would find. She told me the hospital would not admit Beth.

The Case Worker explained that my wife was leaving because the x-ray found no fractures, and there was no reason to keep her. I strongly objected, reasoning that my wife could not walk without tremendous pain. The Case Worker repeated that pain comes with any fall, and she is just experiencing that pain. She told me Home Health Care would be notified and have a nurse come by in the morning to evaluate her to see if she may need physical therapy. I strenuously objected to her leaving, reasoning that if the nurse could not walk her to the bathroom, how would I walk her into the house?

I asked to talk to the doctor but instead got the nurse with the discharge papers to sign.

I only had contact with the doctor when he came by and said, "Good news, no fractures, and he was gone."

The nurse had me sign the discharge papers while placing an ACE bandage on the lower part of Beth's leg, gave her some pain medication, and, with much difficulty, my wife was put in a wheelchair and wheeled out to the parking lot. In excruciating pain, Beth was placed in the car by the two nurses having the same difficulty experienced when putting her in the wheelchair.

During the four hours in the ER, Beth was never checked to see if she could put weight on her left leg without a walker or asked to take a step without assistance. Before discharge, a nurse's 'road test' is the final say on whether the patient can leave.

If there is doubt, the nurse must notify the doctor that the patient failed the 'road test' so the doctor can reevaluate his decision to discharge the patient. Beth's final discharge medical advice came from the ER nurse and the Case Worker, and at no time was she told not to load bear on the leg until she saw an orthopedic doctor nor given a 'road test' as previously defined.

After gingerly putting Beth onto the car's front seat, we left for the fifteen-minute drive home, still in tremendous pain. Getting home, I got her a walker and, despite her pain complaints, managed to get her out of the car. She took five steps from the car to a five-inch step at the house entrance. When she took the step, putting total weight on the injured leg, she collapsed into a sitting position in the doorway.

She did not fall but collapsed like a building if you removed the side walls. She was in tremendous pain, and there was no way I could lift her to a standing position to get her to her walker and into the house. My only alternative was to make a 911 call for lifting help.

EMS arrived and got her to her feet but could not get her from the doorway to the bathroom since she could not walk. They asked for a wheeled desk chair, and she was placed on it and pushed to the toilet. When done, they got her seated, put her back on the chair, and wheeled her to bed. Every time she was moved, she complained about the excruciating pain.

I asked what to do if she had to go to the bathroom at night, and EMS told me to use the desk chair to get her to the toilet and, if I could not get her up, to call EMS again for lift help. At 4:00 AM, she had to go to the bathroom. I got her on the chair and the toilet seat, and, as expected, I could not stand her up to get her back onto the chair. As recommended, I again called 911 for EMS lift help.

They arrived shortly and brought her back into bed despite much pain. They looked at her leg, swollen to about one and half times its standard size, was black and blue and hard as a rock. They said the leg did not look good, and she belonged in the hospital. I informed them she had just been discharged from the ER, who informed us there was nothing broken, and the pain and swelling were the after-effects of the fall. EMS told me I was in an inconvenient situation since she had a problem, but whom do you go to if the hospital tells you there is nothing wrong because they could find no fractures?

After a sleepless night in the morning, I removed the ACE bandage applied in the ER, thinking it may shut off the blood supply and cause swelling. The leg was black, and she was in pain every time she moved her leg. I called Home Health Care to see how quickly they could get one of their nurses to look at my wife's leg. Calling them was what the Case Worker told me to do, having informed me she would send a referral to Home Health at once.

Much to my surprise, Home Health told me they had no referral for my wife and would need a referral from the hospital before sending anyone over. I informed them I had a referral, but they told me the protocol required Home Health to receive a referral from the hospital before they could open a case. I said I needed someone at once to look at my wife's leg to see whether she should return to the ER. Home Health would check with the hospital and call me right back.

After waiting an hour with no response, I called the ER directly, described my wife's condition, and was informed to get her back to the ER. Once again, a call to 911 brought back the EMS to transport her. EMS arrived, finding her pain was terrible; they moved her from the bed to their stretcher by lifting the sheet she was lying on and moving it to the stretcher.

She arrived at 10:45 AM and remained in the hall on a gurney until 2:00 PM when a doctor finally saw her. He asked why she was there; she showed him her leg and detailed the preceding evening's events. He informed me she needed an ultrasound exam and told me I could go home since it was apparent that she would be admitted.

At 3:00 PM, the hospital called to inform me that the ultrasound revealed she had a fractured tibia and fibula, the two bones in the lower leg, and he would admit her to the hospital. The swelling and bruising were so bad that the surgeon could not operate until both conditions dissipated. Rather than fill a hospital surgical bed, she would be moved to the HPCC skilled nursing facility and remain there until the swelling and bruising had gone down sufficiently to operate, such determination to be made by the surgeon.

With time to think, I asked myself, "Did the ER send my wife home on Friday night with a broken leg?" Studying the tibia on the internet, I concluded Beth had a stable fracture meaning the tibia had a possible hairline fracture that would have been evident with ultrasound when first admitted. Though the x-rays of the hip, pelvis, and knee showed no fractures, her complaint of pain below the knee should have called for an ultrasound.

However, the ER nurse did not inform the doctor of my wife's continued pain complaint and inability to walk. Correcting a cracked and a broken tibia is substantially different, with a break needing surgery and a cracked tibia placed in a brace for a few months to restrict weight bearing until healed. The tibia crack would be why it collapsed as soon as the weight was put on it when Beth tried to enter the house. Question: was the ER guilty of negligence in sending Beth home with a broken leg?

Chapter 2
Rehabilitation

On 18 May, Beth entered the HPCC skilled nursing facility to wait for the swelling to go down enough to operate; the surgeon's determination was to be made on 1 June. She is in constant pain, and all HPCC can do is keep her on prescribed pain medication, which does little to dull the pain. Beth is showing signs of depression and has expressed the desire to die rather than wake up each morning and be in pain for the remainder of the day.

She is in an immobilizer and needs help whenever she urinates. HPCC on 18 May, in violation of Medicare directives about the restricted use of a catheter, unless medically necessary, embedded a urinary catheter, a decision not medically justified, but more as a convenience to the aides to eliminate their need to help her to the bathroom or to change diapers—an important date.

I will briefly mention Medicare's directive about using urinary catheters here and cover it in more detail later. Medicare states, "Ensure a resident who enters the facility without an indwelling catheter is not catheterized unless the resident's clinical condition demonstrates catheterization was necessary, and if the resident subsequently receives one, it is removed as soon as possible." Urinary catheters are the number one cause of urinary tract infections (UTIs).

On 1 June, we discussed her operation with her orthopedic surgeon. The surgeon reviewed the x-rays of her break with us and then gave her unwelcome news. The fracture was more a shatter of the tibia and was so bad that it would be considered significant surgery. Another factor that would make surgery risky is that her bones are so soft due to her having osteoporosis and would not hold the screws necessary to hold the metal plate he would attach.

Because of the substantial risk of surgery failure, he advised not to do the surgery but let the bones heal themselves. He projected the rehab time would be 16 to 19 weeks, and the leg would never be the same. This news sent Beth into significant depression, knowing she would suffer for another five months.

I asked the surgeon to review the x-rays taken on 12 May when she was admitted to the ER to see if he saw any evidence of a tibia break. He studied the X-rays and saw what he thought was an abnormality that may not have been clear to an ER doctor. I asked if this abnormality could have caused the pain she experienced during the so-called 'road test' and if the pain alone should have needed further examination. He agreed that pain alone would have been sufficient reason to admit her to the hospital for an ortho consult or for the ER doctor to have ordered an ultrasound exam in addition to the x-rays.

She should not have left the hospital on 12 May. When asked why she was—he indirectly and off the record—referred to hospital policy to hold down admissions from the ER. If this was true, my wife's foreseeable months of pain might have been dictated by policy rather than medical judgment. The surgeon ordered a full custom-made leg brace that a technician from the manufacturer would fit.

Knowing surgery is not an option for repairing her leg; her depression has become more apparent. She is not eating and has become confused, probably due to the heavy pain medication. Her desire to die needed calling the facility's Quality-of-Life team to treat her depression. Adding to her depression, she is now suffering from a spastic bladder and has the feeling of having to urinate even though she has a catheter. The catheter could cause this feeling, and the urge to pee has become her biggest complaint. She is not eating and spends most of her day sleeping, and her confusion has become more apparent.

On Sunday, 4 June, I got a surprise call from her ortho surgeon, and in the discussion, it became clear he was thinking about this case. He explained what the new brace would do, keeping her leg fixed to allow the bones to grow together. He detailed the ramifications of trying to operate with an extremely high probability of failing.

On 5 June, due to her constant pain complaint and spastic bladder problems, I called her pain management physician and scheduled an appointment. Reviewing her pain medications, he informed us she was getting the most potent drug he would recommend, so there was nothing more he could do for her pain. On 6 June, I talked with Beth's Case Manager, who expressed that the staff is worried about her because she is not eating and has gone downhill from her condition when admitted. I asked the Q Life team to revisit her and make any recommendations.

On 6 June, the representative from the leg brace manufacturer came to measure Beth for the prescribed brace. He spent thirty minutes taking leg measurements which required manipulating the leg. During this excruciating procedure, Beth slept through the whole process, not waking once.

Two days later, the $600, custom-made, complicated brace arrived. It consisted of twelve molded plastic pieces connected by metal bars, four straps to attach the brace to the leg, and many adjusting screws to set it at the correct 30 to 40-degree angle. The angle setting is essential to keep the leg in the proper position to aid healing. The brace representative instructed a physical therapist and me on the appropriate method for attaching the brace and stressed the importance of appropriately securing it. He also noted the importance of being removed daily to check for sores that may develop under the brace.

I immediately recognized there was no possibility that an aide would take the fifteen minutes necessary to remove the mount, check the leg for sores, and then reattach the brace in the prescribed manner. My inclinations became a reality when I returned the following day and found the brace incorrectly attached. Finding no aide or physical therapist available, I reattached the brace myself. Many days after that, I found the brace improperly attached and made the correction myself.

One can have the state-of-the-art leg brace, explicitly designed to ensure proper healing of my wife's fracture. It does not serve its designed purpose if it is continuously incorrectly attached. An additional problem with the brace is that it makes sleeping difficult without being medicated. It limits her sleep positions and now adds sleeplessness to the urinary issues. It also has severely reduced her mobility, and she will depend more on aide assistance.

On 9 June, I talked with the physical therapist, who informed me Beth was not cooperating with them because she always wanted to sleep. The sleep is probably the result of her taking Percocet and Xanax, both sedatives, with the expected outcome being that she wants to sleep. The physical therapist told me she was not making progress; if she did not improve, physical therapy would have to end.

My next question was, "Why is she on physical therapy when she will be in a brace for the next 16 to 19 weeks?"

"Wouldn't it be more practical to start PT when she is weight-bearing on the broken leg?" I learned that even though Beth is in the facility for the long-term care necessary for her leg to heal, HPCC gets paid for sixty days of physical therapy provided there is progress, and if not, Medicare payments stop. So, they are giving her occupational therapy, which is upper body, even though the treatment would have no application until she is out of her brace.

Her confusion has worsened; she is not eating and keeps crying, "I have to pee." Her shouting resulted in her being moved to another room because her roommate complained about her screaming. Her need to urinate with an empty bladder has become her most significant problem, even topping the pain. It has gotten to the point where the staff puts her on the toilet, where she tries her best to urinate with no results.

One day, I got a call; she was unmanageable, had removed her brace, and tried walking to the bathroom. Telling her she has a catheter in does no good since the urge to go is still there. I got an appointment with her urologist to see if he could alleviate this urge to pee.

She is becoming increasingly unmanageable and tries to remove her brace continuously so she can walk to the toilet and pee. I am beginning to wonder whether the urge is physical or psychological. The facility finally had a psych consult to manage her agitation and depression. The doctor prescribed a new antidepressant, and there seems to be some improvement. I even brought in a Scrabble game and played the game with her many times.

Surprisingly, her mind is sound. She figures out words, does the addition, and never once complains about having to pee. Is the question of her need to pee physical or mental? It has gotten so bad that she will ride her wheelchair down the hall, hunting for a bathroom so she can pee. During the day, the nurses keep her at the nurse's station to watch her.

We went to her urologist appointment, hoping he could diagnose her problem.

His first question was, "Why does she have a catheter in rather than be in diapers?" I told him I did not know.

He responded, "I know why; it is convenient for the attendants not to have to change her diaper all the time."

"It is to make their job easier and not for medical necessity."

"The insertion of the catheter for any length of time will drastically increase her susceptibility to urinary tract infection for the rest of her life."

"The catheter may cause her urge to urinate, but it is probably a mental condition with antidepressants being the only means of treatment."

"She feels like she has to urinate, but there is nothing physically wrong with her that can be treated with any medication I may give her," the doctor's diagnosis blows our hopes that the urologist could prescribe something to treat the urge to urinate.

I researched the constant urge to urinate with no physical cause present and produced what I suspected her condition might be. It is a psychosomatic illness with a sub-grouping of Somatic Symptom Disorder or SSD. With SSD, the individual feels the physical symptoms even though no physical cause is clear. It used the example of people experiencing all the cancer symptoms even though they do not have cancer.

Medication cannot cure the illness; one can only treat it. Treatment is mental conditioning, and there are SSD medications that may or may not help. The medicines now given are trying to treat a non-existing physical condition. Doctors do not like to get a diagnosis from those with WebMD credentials, so they ignore my diagnosis.

I explained my SSD diagnosis to Beth and told her she had to mentally get her mind off the urge to pee and concentrate on something else.

For example, when we played Scrabble for an hour or more, she did not say, "I got to pee." She said she understood, but I doubt it will cure her urge to pee.

Beth's continued "I have to pee" mantra and her trying to get out of bed to go to the bathroom required the nurses to respond to her room all night. They moved her to a room near the nurse's station to correct the situation. On 30 June, I noticed she was less agitated and not complaining about having to pee continuously. Per my suggestion, HPCC had put her on Seroquel, an antidepressant that may have helped her. She is now going for hours without needing to pee, so pain is now her major complaint.

I visit her for three hours daily, taking her out on the patio in her wheelchair and playing Scrabble on the terrace or in the game room. I visit around dinnertime, so I can accompany her to get her to eat. I have been called at home many nights to try calming her down when she is experiencing severe pain or pee problems. I will sit with her until she calms down and goes to sleep.

One night I was called in because she was unmanageable, had removed her brace, and was sitting on the commode. No one knows how she got there, and that is one of the attendant's problems; she wants to take off the brace and walk to the bathroom. The constant urge to pee must be excruciatingly painful, and it is heartbreaking to be unable to help her. The other sad request is her asking when she can go home. She wants so badly to go home, and I find diverse ways to tell her she will not go home until she can walk again.

Let me go off script here for an explanation of a Medicare problem. On 14 July 2017, HPCC notified me that Beth's Medicare status would expire on the 17th when she would have to leave or pay $275 a day because her 60 days of physical therapy had progressed as far as possible. My response was that she was not in HPCC for biological treatment but skilled nursing and needed to address the care of the leg brace.

Giving occupational therapy for 60 straight days to a resident who will not be weight-bearing for an unspecified number of weeks seems excessive and a play on Medicare's paying for 60 days of therapy. Medicare pays for 60 days of physical treatment provided the patient shows progress. By giving her PT daily for 60 days and informing Medicare she was progressing, Medicare would pay the facility for the PT. I question how HPCC could tell Medicare Beth was improving during those paid 60 days, but her progression ended on day sixty-one. I appealed to Medicare.

Medicare turned my appeal down. The Decision Explanation states that skilled nursing services may be necessary to improve the patient's condition, which requires the bones to grow together, which therapy cannot improve. To maintain the patient's condition (the leg stabilizing brace supports that state and to prevent further deterioration of the patient's condition again, that is the purpose of the brace, not therapy)."

The decision to deny also said, "Such skilled therapy services are covered when an individualized assessment of the patient's clinical condition demonstrates that a qualified therapist's specialized judgment, knowledge, and skills are necessary for the performance of the rehabilitation services."

Why was physical therapy started on day one and continued for eight weeks knowing the patient could not bear weight on her leg for an unknown period and would thus not meet the Medicare requirements for showing progress? That lack of progress is why Medicare would not grant further Medicare coverage.

The Explanation of the Unfavorable Decision describes the issue as 'skilled nursing facility services.' It also states that to cover post-hospital care in a skilled nursing facility (SNF), Medicare requires patients to receive medically reasonable and necessary skilled nursing daily. Only on an inpatient basis in an SNF can provide that professional service.

"Coverage for skilled therapy inpatient services does not turn on the presence or absence of a beneficiary's potential, but rather on the beneficiary's need for skilled care." If therapy does not turn on potential, how can lack of progress be grounds for discontinuing Medicare coverage for skilled nursing? Beth meets Medicare's criteria for needing 'skilled nursing.'

I also disagreed with the decision, "The medical record does not support she could derive that additional benefit from an SNF level of care for further improvement, restoration or to prevent or slow further deterioration of the beneficiary's current status."

The added benefit derived from the SNF level of care is that the surgeon orders that the leg is checked daily for blood clots or leg sores. Only by ensuring these conditions do not occur can the patient show further improvement as the healing process continues to its conclusion.

I did not send the second appeal to Medicare because it became unnecessary. I noticed that Beth's memory had worsened in the last few days. Beth calls me increasingly at night, telling me she has no idea where she is and asking why she cannot come home. I do not know whether this is dementia or another UTI.

She also appeared dehydrated, so I performed a skin turgor test, which lightly pinches the skin to see how long it takes to bounce back, and determined she was dry. I informed the charge nurse that I believed Beth was dehydrated. The nurse then also did a turgor test and agreed with my diagnosis. She told me they would give her more to drink, but it is evident she is not drinking what they are now giving her, thus resulting in dehydration.

It became evident that the dehydration was worsening, and I informed them that the nurse should put her on an IV to rehydrate her. She agreed and said they would start one. She was not on an IV the next day when I visited. I asked why not and was told the nurses tried to get an IV in four times, but her veins kept collapsing. No staff member could insert the IV line, so they stopped trying and reverted to getting her to take in more fluids. Beth continues to show increased signs of confusion and is lethargic. I went to the PA assigned to the floor and told her Beth's dehydration was worsening, and HPCC needed to send her to the ER. She told me the ER would IV her and send her back.

I said, "If she is dehydrated, rehydration is the purpose of sending her to the hospital."

Rather than rehydrating her in the ER, the facility chose to do nothing. I continued to complain that her BUN level on her blood work was high, which usually shows dehydration. She is not drinking, her skin is not responding to skin turgor testing, and she needs to move to the ER. The nurses were not receptive to my suggestion and told me they would find a nurse who could insert the IV for rehydration at HPCC. Eventually, a nurse, after much difficulty, inserts the IV line. Rehydration started on 27 July, but it became clear that they began the process too late.

On 28 July, Beth had an appointment with her ortho surgeon for an x-ray of the leg to see how it was healing. Surprisingly, the bones knitted well, and the doctor removed the brace. However, the doctor's office nurse noticed Beth was unresponsive and fell asleep in her wheelchair. The nurses had difficulty getting her onto the exam table because she was weak. They recognized there was something here that needed to be addressed by HPCC.

The surgeon wrote a script that Beth could now bear weight on her leg, and rehab could begin. I then discussed with him the failure of the hospital to find the tibia fracture during her initial ER visit. I will address this discussion later. Upon return to the HPCC, I gave the nurse's station the doctor's script showing her now being in a weight-bearing status for rehab. When I left her, all she wanted to do was sleep, and again, I told the staff she was dehydrated.

On Saturday, 29 July, I received a call at home from HPCC telling me they found Beth in a non-responsive state and were putting her on an IV awaiting the facility doctor's arrival. Another call two hours later informed me that HPCC had rushed Beth to the ER. When I arrived at the ER, the doctors were in aggressive rehydration, and she was still non-responsive. Into the second bag of saline solution, she finally came around.

In addition, she was diagnosed with a UTI and pneumonia, and the hospital admitted her. The UTI and dehydration were probably the cause of her confusion. HPCC called wanting to know what to do with her belongings, and I said to leave them there since I was expecting her to return after hospital discharge.

The case Manager on 1 August informed me Beth was to be discharged from the hospital and wanted to know what facility she was going to. I said to return her to HPCC, the facility that sent her to the hospital, only to have the

Case Manager tell me they had no bed for her. A bed hold form, as required, was to be sent by HPCC with her hospital admission forms, but HPCC still needs a document. The bed hold form informs me I could hold the bed by paying a $ 100-bed hold fee for the days she was hospitalized, which I would have gladly paid.

The Case Manager, off the record, told me she heard HPCC did not want her back because she required too much attendant care. So, after spending eleven weeks in rehab, and now when effective rehab therapy could begin, they no longer want her. Not readmitting a resident is a practice AARP refers to as nursing home eviction and is a practice AARP has filed suit against.

The Case Worker and I searched for another rehab facility with an available bed. One was found, but it was like going from the Hilton to Motel 6, and it was different from the one I would have chosen if choices were available. HPCC, being part of the hospital system, could employ experienced staff by paying good wages with benefits. The new facility, which I will refer to as FMR, was primarily staffed with aides from Haiti or Jamaica.

They were good people, but the experience needed to be improved due to the high turnover of aides. Beth at once noticed the change in environment and became even more depressed. She has only thirty days left on Medicare for room and board and physical therapy. Medicare physical therapy payments begin again after a recipient spends three days in a hospital.

On 13 August, I stopped by FMR to see how her physical therapy was going and found them doing only upper body therapy and not concentrating on getting her mobile. I asked why physical therapy was not focused on getting her walking again and was told, according to the hospital discharge documents, that she was non-weight bearing. I informed them she had been weight-bearing since 28 July.

A review of the hospital documents shows her to be non-weight bearing, and the hospital records reflect what was given to them by HPCC when sending Beth to the ER. FMR informed me she was sent to the ER by HPCC with incorrect information by not including the doctor's orders for her to be weight-bearing. When I requested a copy of the transfer to the ER documents from HPCC, the facility refused. Either HPCC or the hospital transferring incorrect patient status information resulted in Beth not getting ten days of desperately needed weight-bearing exercises, leaving her only 15 days of PT remaining.

At FMR, she continued complaining about having to pee even though the catheter was embedded. The head nurse asked me why she had the catheter. I told him I knew of no medical reason, and her urologist believed it was strictly for the convenience of HPCC's aides so they would not have to change diapers or help her to the bathroom. The urologist determined there was no medical problem requiring a catheter. The nurse also informed me of Beth's difficulties urinating once the catheter is out. It had been in over two months, and her bladder had been inactive for that period, and the muscles would have weakened.

Like her urologist, he also informed me she would be subject to frequent urinary tract infections for the rest of her life. I told him I knew all the pitfalls associated with catheters, but I had to assume HPCC embedded the catheter for medical reasons. He asked whether I objected to his removing it since we both decided there was no medical reason for the catheter to remain. The catheter had been in for an estimated 90 days when taken out.

It was at this point that I researched the use of catheters. Every website, including Medicare's, emphasizes that catheters be embedded only if medically necessary. If required, a catheter should be removed as soon as possible because of the known side effects of urinary tract infections. I first thought HPCC might have been guilty of medical misconduct with their use of a catheter not justified by medical necessity.

On 16 August, 97 days after breaking her tibia, I reviewed her condition. She is in constant pain from the physical therapy and still frequently urges to pee, even though FMR has removed the catheter. She is becoming more depressed and has again expressed the desire to die rather than suffer the debilitating daily pain with no end.

She can dress with the brace removed, but she is still not eating and has lost eleven pounds. She has no idea when the bones will mend but knows she will be in constant pain until they do. Medicare expires in fifteen days, and she has to be able to graduate to home health PT or pay a $300 per day charge to remain at the facility.

On 28 August, her Medicare days had elapsed, and she left FMC to begin physical therapy at home. She is glad to leave because the nursing home environment makes her more depressed. She was surrounded by many others in wheelchairs, many in declining health, knowing many would never leave the nursing home. She is still coming home a long way from walking without pain and experiencing the frequent urge to pee.

In summary, her rehab has done little to get her back to her condition before her fall, and I have acknowledged that she will never regain the quality of life she had before her fall. She now faces physical therapy two and three days a week at home. A few days before leaving FMR, she fell and severely bruised her tailbone, a severe injury. I requested that FMR send her to the ER, but they discouraged doing so since she would be leaving rehab in a few days, and if necessary, I could take her to the ER.

I did, and the hospital admitted her for intractable back pain. She spent five days in the hospital, where they were unsuccessful in reducing the pain. The doctor informed her that a bruised tailbone was painful and would not heal for up to two years. The medical profession could do nothing outside of pain medication, and the bruising would eventually heal.

She will start rehab physical therapy three days a week at home administered by a Home Health Agency. Even though the therapist spends most of her time filling out reports, she manages to give her a good workout in the hour she is working with Beth. Beth will never walk again without a walker, and I worry about her falling when I am not home. I now started thinking about her going to assisted living.

Chapter 3
CMS 20068

Thinking I might have a medical malpractice claim, I researched the internet to find an applicable regulation governing the use of an embedded catheter. I found the Holy Grail, a rule that solidified my belief that I had a lawsuit. The principle is detailed here and will be referred to as CMS 20068 in the story.

Title: URINARY CATHETER OR URINARY TRACT INFECTION CRITICAL ELEMENT PATHWAY issued by the Department of Health and Human Services Center for Medicare Services. Form CMS 20068.

Critical Element Decisions:

Based on observations, interviews, and records review, did the facility provide excellent and sufficient services, treatment, and care, based upon current standards of practice and the resident's comprehensive assessment and care plan to:

Ensure a resident who enters the facility without an indwelling catheter is not catheterized unless the resident's clinical condition shows catheterization was necessary;

Ensure a resident who enters the facility with an indwelling catheter or later receives one is assessed for removal of the catheter as soon as possible unless the resident's clinical condition proves catheterization is necessary; and

Ensure a resident receives proper treatment and services to prevent urinary tract infections.

Has staff involved the resident or representative in developing a care plan, including whether interventions reflect preferences and choices, and discussed the risks and benefits of a urinary catheter? Failure of HPCC to observe the mandates of Medicare about using an indwelling catheter will be the basis for our medical malpractice lawsuit. HPCC, being a Medicare facility, is required to observe these mandates.

Chapter 4
Malpractice Case

There could be grounds for filing a lawsuit supported by off-the-record discussions with Beth's ortho surgeon. Based on our conversations, I extrapolated the following statements:

A review of the original x-ray taken of Beth's left knee showed what appeared to be an abnormality present on the left side of the knee. The exception and the complaint of pain below her knee could indicate a stable tibia fracture. Based on the knee x-ray abnormality and her pain criticism, she should not have been discharged from the ER on 12 May. If a standard 'road test' had been performed before Beth was released, it would have substantiated his contention that she should not have been discharged.

When Beth placed her total body weight on the left leg when entering the house, the possible, stable fracture became a multi-fracture of the tibia. He reviewed the statements and agreed they could be factual but would not sign off on them because he has to work with this community. I agreed with his position and reluctance to sign off.

Convinced there was a valid malpractice suit against the hospital, I reviewed the nursing home's actions to see if I had documentation to pursue a case against HPCC. I called the Administrator of HPCC to inform him.

On 29 July, HPCC notified me they had sent my wife, in a non-responsive state, to the hospital emergency room due to severe dehydration, a condition I recognized and reported several times to the HPCC nursing staff. Agreeing that Beth was dehydrated, they would start a rehydration IV. Upon returning to the facility and not finding my wife on an IV, I asked the charge nurse why not. She responded that the staff tried to insert an IV, but her veins kept collapsing, so they discontinued their efforts and rehydrate her by having her drink more.

My blood work review showed her BUN level continuing to escalate, and I informed the charge nurse that she needed to be sent to the ER for rehydration. After our discussion, a nurse could insert an IV feeding line and start an IV drip, but it appeared it was too late. She was rushed to the ER three days later, dehydrated and non-responsive. Dehydration was a condition the facility was aware of but chose to ignore.

He responded, "I will review the actions of the staff."

Upon discharge from the hospital, I was told by the Case Manager that she would not be returning to HPCC because they no longer had a bed for her, and I would have to find a rehab facility elsewhere. A call to the nursing supervisor to inquire why Beth was not returning referred me to the bed hold policy.

Notice upon transfer—upon patient transfer out of the facility; nursing will supply a copy of HPCC's Bed Hold Policy in the transfer packet and contact the patient or patient representative to discuss the Bed Hold Policy. The Business Office will contact the patient or representative the next business day to complete the bed hold stratus.

I told him HPCC never contacted me as per the policy, and if HPCC had sent a bed hold form with the patient, I would have been given the form by the Case Manager. She told me no bed hold form came with Beth and asked if the facility had contacted me about how to ensure her bed would be held for her return. I assured her I had not been approached and assumed she would return there since she transferred out of HPCC due to their negligence.

The final word was that the facility would not take her back, and my only choice was to find another facility. This new facility would know very little of her condition or procedures done in the last seventy days at HPCC. The administrator said the facility followed all the Bed Hold Policies, and he would review it further to see if they could improve the notification process. I then asked him to send me a copy of the records that went with Beth to the ER from HPCC on 29 July to see if a bed hold policy form went with the documents. He said he would not grant my request for a copy of the transferred records.

I received a letter from HPCC's Administrator and Risk Manager, who said I received the bed hold form. I told her I never got the document because, per the hospital Case Manager, no record came with Beth's transfer to the hospital, violating HPCC's Bed Hold Policy. She insisted that the staff notified me.

I repeated that the only notification I got was "What do you want to do with Beth's clothing?" which I replied to hold at the facility, assuming she would be returning. She said I had declined to sign a bed hold form, which was false since it would have been foolish for me not to sign the paper since she had just spent seventy days at the facility. By not signing the form, I would have to have another rehab lined up to receive her upon hospital discharge, which I did not have.

A copy of the transferring forms I requested would have shown whether a bed hold form, per facility policy, would have been included and whether the hospital knew Beth was now weight-bearing. This information would tell me if HPCC was negligent in not sending a bed hold form and not informing the hospital that Beth was now weight-bearing for physical therapy.

Reviewing the actions of the hospital and the nursing home, I decided I had enough data to prepare a malpractice suit and prepared the following summary of my conclusions. I contend that the medical staff at the hospital emergency room was derelict in their duties about administering adequate medical care on 12 May 2017 by not finding a broken tibia. My contention is based on the following procedures or lack thereof.

The ER discharged my wife after a fall at home when x-rays revealed no bone fractures above the knee, even though she complained of severe pain and could not walk without pain. Failure of the ER discharge nurse to perform an adequate "'road test' on my wife, as requested by the doctor, was a contributing factor to her injury. Despite much pain, the test consisted of my wife standing, supported by a walker. A request from me, the nurse walk her to the bathroom to see if she could walk without pain, was ignored.

The medical description of a 'road test' states: "The test assesses discharge suitability criteria by the testing level of self-sufficiency, cerebellar function gait, ataxia, ambulation, and the ability to understand discharge instructions."

"Ambulation is the ability to walk from place to place independently with or without assistive devices."

The Case Manager met my repeated emphasis that my wife could not walk without pain, repeating, "The pain is just the expected result of the fall."

The nurse again ignored my request to see the doctor. There is no mention in the discharge instructions informing my wife not to weigh bear on the leg until she sees her doctor, and the ER nurse's failure to give such instructions resulted in my wife collapsing when she placed weight on the injured leg. She collapsed and did not fall, as the ER readmittance information said.

My contention, as supported by the opinion of her ortho surgeon, is that my wife had a possible, stable tibia fracture, which would have been found with an ultrasound, preventing it from becoming a shattered tibia when she put weight thereon. The performance of a proper 'road test' would have shown that my wife did not meet the standard ambulation criteria of the test, and the nurse should have notified the doctor. Informing the doctor would have flagged the possibility of a fracture below the knee, and he could have ordered x-rays below the knee or asked for an orthopedic consult.

I contend that an ultrasound of the lower leg would have shown the suspected stable tibia fracture before it became a broken, shattered tibia. A stable fracture would have required the leg to be immobilized for a period, but the rehab would have been at home and not in a skilled nursing facility. The tibia shattering resulted in massive swelling and bruising, evident twenty days after the incident when reviewed by her orthopedic surgeon. She spent those twenty days in a skilled nursing facility on huge painkilling medication, which provided little relief.

My contention, supported by the orthopedic surgeon, is that my wife should never have been discharged from the ER without further examination of her leg when she complained of continued pain. We believe the tibia was fractured at the time of discharge. In summary, the failure of the ER at the hospital to conduct a proper 'road test' before discharging my wife has resulted in subjecting her to months of debilitating pain in a skilled nursing facility and the possibility of permanent damage to her future mobility. Because of their negligence, the hospital should be held liable for their actions.

Case Summary: The hospital emergency room did not administer a standard 'road test,' despite many requests to do so, before discharging my wife, who, shortly after discharge, collapsed when exiting the car upon arriving home. She was later readmitted to the ER with a shattered, inoperable tibia/fibula fracture. As a result of the ER's neglect, my wife will spend the next four to five months in extremely painful rehab with severe leg damage that would have been evident if a standard one-minute 'road test' had been performed before her discharge. In summary, the hospital sent my wife home with a broken leg.

I sent this summary to several attorneys, thinking I would be fine getting a firm to discuss this case. How wrong I was to be.

Chapter 5
The Plaintiffs

On 15 August 1936, Beth was born in Akron, Ohio, but grew up on a western Pennsylvania farm. Her mother was a retired RN, and her father managed a meat processing plant in town. Upon graduating high school, she entered the nurses' training program at Columbia Hospital in Pittsburg, a three-year, in-hospital training program, with her living in the hospital dorm. It was while she was still in training that she met me. After serving three years on a US Navy destroyer with two tours of duty in Korea, I attended Duquesne University on the GI bill. I was only 23 years old, joining the Navy right out of high school at seventeen.

Along with my friends, I heard of a bar where nurses spent time together, so we decided to try our luck. That is where we met, and even though I was not the one she wanted to go home with, I was the one who got to take her back to her dorm. We hit it off, and the rest is history.

She graduated in 1957 and went right into her chosen nursing desire, being an operating room nurse. She became so good at her duties that she became one of the few nurses doctors asked for by name to aid them in surgery.

I graduated in 1958 and took a job with Dan River Mills in Danville, Virginia. The assignment resulted in a long-distance relationship with my getting back, after an eight-hour drive, about once a month. I spent only nine months in Danville before moving on to a new job in Montgomery, Alabama, as a plant industrial engineer, thus extending our long-distance relationship beyond driving distance.

Wedding plans were already made, and on 1 August 1959, we were married and at once packed a trailer and attached it to a car her father gave us and headed for Montgomery. We married on a Saturday, and I had to return to work the following Tuesday. We spent our wedding night in a run-down motel in Cincinnati, Ohio.

Montgomery was quite a change for both of us. Being northern Catholics, we did not fit into the setting. Being a Yankee was terrible, but being Catholic was foreign to the Southern Baptists. Beth at once got a job in the hospital's ER department, working the 3 to 11 evening shifts. This job ended after she was followed home one night after work and ran scared into the house. She then entered the new field of industrial nursing when I got her the post in the plant where I worked.

The employees liked her, and the nurses' station became popular. On the Easter holidays from work in 1960, we decided to take a honeymoon trip to New Orleans. During the drive down, Beth experienced what was not her only miscarriage. It occurred in a service station restroom and was quite traumatic for us.

We enjoyed our time in Montgomery, where we bought our first home, a yellow brick ranch with pink shutters. It cost all of $13,000, a fortune at that time. Especially since I graduated from college and worked at my first job, I was paid $70 a week for a 45-hour week. I moved to my new job at the increased salary of $412 a month, so a $13,000 expenditure was quite a bit, but we could meet the mortgage payments with both of us working.

We also learned about the Southern view of segregation; even though I experienced it in Danville, this was Beth's first experience. She had an excellent rapport with the women of color working in the plant when the whites looked down upon them. Many employees resented her treatment of the 'colored folks.' Our exposure to Montgomery's view of the colored occurred one Sunday.

The Reverend Abernathy, a cohort of Dr. Martin Luther King, announced that the blacks would do a demonstration march on the capitol building protesting discrimination practices of the city government. So, from a church in their Sunday best clothing, hundreds of folks gathered outside the church where the demonstration was to originate. At 2:00, when the march began, the protesters started down from the church, and the crowd started to beat them up and throw objects at them.

I noticed four Allied Van Line trailers parked near the capitol building, and when the riot started, the doors on those trailers opened, and horse-mounted state troopers rode into the crowd with long sticks in their hand and started swinging to break up the public. Next, the fire department arrived and hosed down the group to break up the riot. The blacks then retreated into the church; eventually, everyone went home. I was taking pictures of the event when accosted by one of the rioters who wanted to know if I was 'one of those Yankee newspaper photographers.' I convinced him I was just another Alabama red-neck in my best southern accent, and he moved on.

In Montgomery, we got our first dog. I went to the local dump to dispose of some trash, and this puppy was in the garbage. I decided to bring it home and surprise Beth. It was the first of many. Our stay in Montgomery ended in November of 1960 when I was laid off and started a new job search.

One of the companies that I sent resumes to was RJ Reynolds Tobacco in Winston-Salem, North Carolina. In summary, I listed my job experience with Dan River. The Director of Industrial Engineering at Dan River was a good friend of the Director of IE at RJR. He gave me an excellent recommendation, and RJR immediately hired me in December 1960. We sold the house in Montgomery and moved into a second-floor rental in Winston Salem with a family with a kennel in the backyard that would house Hooker, our dog.

The dog house had a light bulb burning all the time to heat the home. One night, the bulb slipped off its bracket, dropped into the straw on the dog house floor, and set it on fire. We got the dogs out and could extinguish the fire without calling the fire department. The new dog house did not have indoor heating.

With industrial nursing experience, Beth got a plant nurse job in the main cigarette manufacturing plant. Once again, she became extremely popular with the employees, especially the blacks knowing she was a Yankee. Beth was a smoker, and they always brought her cigarette packs right off the line. I remember the first day she started work.

She got on the interstate highway and, with her poor sense of direction, turned right and not left and was on her way to Greensboro, North Caroline, before realizing she was going the wrong way. Again, we experienced segregation, but now the restrooms were integrated, which was a big step forward for RJR. I was still called a Yankee, but I kept telling people I had to travel north to get to North Caroline, having come from Alabama.

We bought our second home for the increased sum of $33,000. It was a brick ranch; all homes in Winston Salem were brick since the clay in North Caroline was great for making brick and thus were cheap. The house was in the country, and we depended on a well for water. A month before leaving the rental, the husband of the couple had a heart attack. I heard the wife scream and ran downstairs to find him on the floor, non-responsive. I did my best at artificial respiration, but he died when the EMTs arrived.

During our stay in Winston-Salem, Beth had her second miscarriage, which sent her into a bad state of depression with the side effects of becoming anorexic. We started all the tests to see why she could not get pregnant and found no known risk factors. We now turned our thoughts to adoption and inquired through the Catholic Agency in town. They thoroughly investigated our background; the intense questioning made Beth's state of mind even worse.

Before we reached the final stages of adoption, I was offered a promotion and transfer to a Del Monte plant in Lockport, NY, just outside of Buffalo, a fantastic opportunity. It would be only three hours from her home and four hours from mine, so I accepted. In February of 1969, we sold the house and moved.

By this time, we had gone through four dogs and bought what we thought to be a pure-bred basset hound. However, when we took it to the vet, he informed us it was not a basset but a mix. Shortly after that, the people we bought it from told us the mother was a pure basset hound, but the father was not, but he did come from a good neighborhood.

Not able to keep a dog in our new rental apartment in Lockport, we dropped it off at her parent's house on the way north. Her father later informed us that we neglected to tell him the dog was pregnant, which we did not know. However, the dog being part basset, he had no trouble getting rid of the puppies.

We bought a house in Lockport, and Beth started working as a school nurse, a new entry on her resume. I became the plant manager in a few years, and Beth began a new nursing field in geriatrics. Once again, after a quick trip to the ER, Beth had her third miscarriage. Her depression and other problems accelerated, and we gave up on having children. Then miracles of all miracles, at the age of 42 and 45, she became pregnant, and this one was a keeper, born in July of 1978, but it was not an easy birth.

I got the call at work and rushed home to get her to the hospital, almost having a wreck on the way. After a few hours of labor, she moved to the delivery room, and I joined them. The birth started, and I saw the doctor who had trouble with the delivery. I knew there were significant problems when the nurse got up on Beth's stomach, trying to push the baby out.

After delivery, we looked at the baby, a boy, and the nurse took him out of the delivery room. We later found out the umbilical cord was wrapped around the baby's neck, and he aspirated. After a day in intensive care, the baby was fine, and he went home with us on time.

However, Beth's medical problems continued. We scheduled a holiday trip to Hawaii over the Thanksgiving holidays of 1981, and Beth had a doctor's appointment two weeks before. He found a lump on her breast, and a mastectomy was performed and told her chemo would start the following week.

She elected not to do chemo until we returned from Hawaii. She did her exercises on the islands, and we had a wonderful time, even knowing she would start chemo upon her return. Months of weekly chemo and wearing a cold cap to prevent hair loss went fine; thirty years later, she was still cancer-free.

Medical problems did not end there, for she went to her doctor in the summer of 1953 feeling extremely sick. She walked in the front door of the doctor's office, exited in an ambulance, and was rushed to the hospital, where her temperature went to 108 degrees.

When I saw her the next day, she was packed in ice in the intensive care unit, where she remained for three days. She remained in the hospital for three months with a low-grade fever, but the medical profession, including every specialty available, could not determine the cause of her illness. She was finally discharged home, where the fever broke, and she never experienced the symptoms again.

After 25 years of fighting the Buffalo winters, we became snowbirds. We went to Florida for vacations for many years and, in 1996, bought a condominium in Ft Myers. Being a golfer, I found the area to have one of the only courses you could walk, which became the deciding factor for where we would live. Beth was a charge nurse on a nursing home's 3 to 11 shift, overseeing 25 Alzheimer's patients. Little did we know then that this nursing facility would enter our lives again. Later, she also volunteered to work for hospice sitting with dying patients.

Chapter 6
Hip Surgery Lawsuit

Beth started having trouble with her left hip replacement, and the doctor determined that the hip replacement needed to be replaced. The operation went fine, and she was placed in bed with a Velcro-connected stabilizer to keep her leg in place. During the night, she kept calling the nurse to tell her she had much pain in her leg. The traveling nurse unfamiliar with hip replacement surgery would give her pain medication rather than do the obvious, loosen the Velcro, and reattach it.

It was evident to Beth that the leg was swelling, and the nurse needed to relieve the restraint. When the doctor came in the morning, he blew his stack when Beth complained about the pain, and he saw the nurse had not loosened the restraint. It was too late, and Beth had suffered severe nerve damage to her foot. It was readily apparent that I had a valid hospital malpractice case. Being a novice, thinking that I could file a complaint with the hospital and work out a settlement, I sent the following letter to the hospital administrator.

Re: Formal Complaint—Post Operative Nursing Care: On 19 October 1999, Dr. Smith (not his real name here) performed my hip revision surgery at LM Hospital. At 3:00 PM, I was transferred from recovery to a room to begin the recovery period. Shortly after arrival, I complained about the pain I was having in the leg in the immobilizer. The pain increased as the day progressed, and the nurse on duty informed the head nurse. She treated me with the pain medication ordered.

Later in the evening, I told the duty nurse that the pain in my leg had increased, and my foot was numb and cold. She touched my foot and said it did not feel cold. The pain and numbness continued throughout the night, and I informed the duty nurse of my discomfort. At 6:30 AM the following morning, Dr. Smith was told of the pain and numbness in my foot. His assistant immediately removed the immobilizer, and the pain let up, but the numbness did not.

When the numbness continued for the next few days, Dr. Smith called in a neurology consult. He diagnosed the problem as nerve damage, likely caused by the leg immobilizer being too tight for an extended period. From my experience in the nursing profession, I learned that restraints were to be loosed every two hours and readjusted to account for swelling that may occur.

When a patient complains about an extremity feeling cold and numb, it is a sign that circulation to that extremity has decreased. When I complained of pain, numbness, and a cold foot, the immobilizer should have been loosened, the circulation checked, and the immobilizer reapplied. The duty nurse followed none of these procedures. The nurse did not readjust the immobilizer from the time of application on 19 October until its removal on 20 October.

I am now experiencing extreme pain in my foot accompanied by numbness, restricting my hip replacement therapy and recovery. Successful hip revision surgery may have been jeopardized by poor judgment in post-operative nursing care—namely, the failure to loosen the immobilizer when I complained about the pain. Dr. Smith also agrees with the neurologist that the tightness of the immobilizer was the probable cause of the nerve damage.

He is optimistic that the damaged nerves will regenerate and has been prescribed vitamin B6 and prescription drugs to accelerate the process. However, three weeks after surgery, the pain and numbness persist. This formal complaint is sent to be on record about my dissatisfaction with the post-operative nursing care received at the hospital. Further action will depend on the expected nerve regeneration within a reasonable time after my hip replacement rehabilitation.

How dumb I thought the above letter would get the hospital to discuss a settlement. I got a letter from the administrator thanking me for the letter and said they would investigate the complaint. It then became apparent that I needed professional help.

I contacted a local malpractice attorney and described the situation using the above letter to detail the incident. He said I had a case, but he could not take it because Dr. Smith was his friend. He referred me to an attorney in Tampa, who gladly accepted the case. So, on 21 February 2001, a claim was filed against LM Hospital.

To further support the pain and suffering my wife was going through, I kept a post-op chronology running from 19 October through 29 January 2000. Reading this chronology, you can realize the pain and suffering of nerve pain. On 28 October, I made the first call to Dr. Smith, telling him how severe her pain was, and he prescribed the drug Neurontin, a seizure drug found to be helpful in nerve stimulation. There was no letup in the pain, and while doing her walking exercises, she had no feeling in her foot; it felt like it had gone to sleep.

I called the doctor and informed him the pain was just as severe, and he increased the medication dosage. He was optimistic that the nerve would regenerate and asked that he continue to be updated. Her pain continues through the night, making sleep difficult. When she walked with her shoes on, she experienced a stabbing pain that continued throughout the day without letting up.

It now becomes evident that she is suffering from severe depression. She was looking forward to her hip surgery to eliminate the pain she was suffering in her hip before replacement surgery. She is afraid she has just exchanged her hip pain for an even worse foot nerve pain. She increasingly depends on pain pills to get her through the day; the medications only reduce the pain and do not end it.

Dr. Smith keeps telling her the nerve will regenerate, but he also worries. He said he had never experienced anything like this before and had performed over 8000 hip replacement surgeries. Her debilitating pain never disappeared, and she was sent to a neurologist for an NCV nerve test trip to Dr. Smith shows the hip surgery was successful, but the NCV test shows she did suffer nerve damage. He feels the sensory nerve will regenerate, but experience has demonstrated recovery at the rate of about one inch per month.

Her nerve damage extends for eighteen inches, meaning she faces a minimum of eighteen months of continued nerve pain. In a visit to the neurologist, and without our asking, he said Beth had sustained nerve damage caused by the immobilizer being on too tight. He said he could do nothing to correct the nerve damage since only nature could repair the damage, and all he could do was try to control the pain.

I could go on and on about what Beth suffered from the nerve pain resulting from hospital malpractice, but I will just cut to the litigation of the hip replacement lawsuit.

LAWSUIT SETTLEMENT

The case begins with our attorney collecting all the nursing notes for the days in question and the hospital attorney fighting us at every step. In 2001, my wife was called in for a recorded deposition lasting over an hour. The depo terrified her, not knowing what to expect and whether she could answer all the questions correctly. She did okay, but having to do this again scared her. The hospital attorney then subjected Dr. Smith and us to a deposition.

The doctor supported our contention that the nursing staff did not follow his protocol, resulting in nerve damage. In addition, we had a letter from the neurologist, whom Dr. Smith called in to evaluate Beth's nerve damage, whose impression said, "Left peroneal neuropathy—most probably secondary to compression from immobilizer."

We had our case, with the next step being a court-ordered mediation meeting of the plaintiff and the defendant's attorneys. We waited for the hospital attorney to get a mediation date. We left for Buffalo in June of 2002, and in July, we were notified that the session had been scheduled for August, meaning we would now have to fly back to attend the session.

Mediation is for that purpose, but it is a farce. I will describe the complete process later applicable to our present lawsuit. We asked for $200,000; the opposing attorney then went into another room where they probably watched television for fifteen minutes and returned with a $10,000 counteroffer. There is a mediator, making $600 an hour with a three-hour minimum, going from room to room with each party's proposals and responses.

The negotiation finally got down to our asking for a settlement of X and the hospital offering Y. Mediated settlements are confidential, so I cannot present numbers, but payment was in the high five figures. It now came down to whether we wanted to go to trial to try and get more or accept their offer. Being terrified of going to trial, Beth agreed to take the hospital's offer.

The release stated, "for consideration of Y, the receipt and sufficiency thereof acknowledged, the undersigned now release and forever discharge LM hospital and continue with legalese." After contingency fees and expenses, Y was reduced by $28,408. No money will ever compensate her for her suffering and the pain she had to look forward to until the nerve regenerated.

Chapter 7
Search for Attorney

I started searching for a law firm adverting as being skilled in medical malpractice. My first inquiry was to the MM law firm, which advertises they will get you the best settlement. Their motto on television at least five times a day is "MM for the People."

I said, "What the hell?" I am a people, so I called them. My call went through to a secretary who inquired what I was calling about, and I told her it was a medical malpractice case. She asked who the defendant was, and I told her it was the hospital. She said she would check with an attorney and, in two minutes, was back, informing me the firm was not interested in the case. Why was I not one of MM's people? I soon learned they were not against me, the people, but against the not to be mentioned word 'hospital.' MM did not even offer me my free consultation as advertised.

I got a name from the attorney service and sent my case description. After waiting for a response for two weeks, I started a new search. Using the definition of Beth's case, I started with the internet, limiting it to practices in the immediate area. Surprisingly, none of the firms were interested in pursuing the case once they found out it involved a lawsuit against the hospital. I then spread out to the state of Florida and found the same response, either by their rejecting the case on the phone or just not responding to my inquiry.

I managed to interview a local attorney personally and discussed the case with him and an attorney specializing in malpractice suits. They declined the issue and sent me a letter explaining why. Following are portions of that letter.

Thank you for contacting our office about your wife's potential medical malpractice inquiry. As we discussed when we met, legislation enacted in Florida over the last few years, as a direct result of the lobbying efforts of physicians, has made us narrow the range of cases we can accept. These laws enormously increase the costs and time that lawyers must invest in proceeding with any medical negligence investigation or litigation. In addition, our laws require the patient to prove by expert witnesses that the defendant's case was below the prevailing standard of care that other doctors would provide.

In your wife's case, we agree that the emergency room physician should not have discharged her when told she could not walk without pain. However, secondly, and sometimes with more difficulty, we must prove that this departure from the standard of care was the cause, directly or indirectly, of the injuries the patient claims resulting from treatment.

In your wife's case, the injuries sustained resulted from the fall, which brought her to the emergency room in the first place, not the failure of the staff to admit her to the hospital timely. Information obtained on your wife's cases has been considered against the legal requirements described above and from our experience in past cases. We have concluded that her case does not meet our present criteria for recommending further action. As a result, we cannot undertake her representation in these matters.

Please understand that this should not be construed as a sign that no merit exists for her potential claims. This decision is the opinion of our offices only, and you have the right to and should consider consulting other counsel.

I decided to continue searching for other counsel based on the last recommendation. In my search and research, I discovered the major drawback of entering a lawsuit against a hospital. It can be summed up by 'Florida's Sovereign Immunity Statutes.' Following is a summary of those statutes.

Chapter 8
Sovereign Immunity

Sovereign immunity is associated with the idea that the 'King can do no wrong.'

It is an ancient principle based on the idea that the courts had no authority to impose judgments or verdicts on the king because a king established the courts. Sovereign immunity is a legal doctrine that protects a sovereign body, in this case, the hospital and nursing home, which are considered state agencies, from being held liable for civil torts committed by its agencies unless consent to be sued is expressly granted by the sovereign body.

Tort law seeks accountability when parties engage in negligent conduct and aims to compensate the victims. Sovereign immunity is an exception to tort law and gives individuals acting as sovereign entities complete protection against tort liability.

Government immunity was adopted when Justice Oliver Wendell Holmes declared in 1907, "A sovereign is exempt from suit because there can be no legal right as against the authority that makes the law on which the right depends." In other words, since it makes the law, it is not subject to it, thus removing the fairness of the law. In a 1945 Supreme Court opinion, the Court declared sovereign immunity is 'embodied in the Constitution.'

Still, no legal scholars have been able to find where precisely in the constitution this doctrine is 'embodied.' In Marbury vs. Madison in 1803, it was held that "the very essence of civil liberty certainly consists of the right of every individual to claim the protection of the laws whenever he receives an injury." Despite this statement, states are enacting increasingly restrictive laws concerning damage limits.

Florida tried ending sovereign immunity in 1969, but after one year, pressure from school boards and insurance companies compelled lawmakers to resort to it partially. Many lawyers refer to sovereign immunity as the 'Free Kill Law.' Medical negligence injures affect over one million Americans yearly and is the third leading cause of death in the US, surpassed only by cancer and heart disease. So-called 'public' hospitals protected by sovereign immunity are supported partially by taxpayer dollars, yet they receive millions in private insurance annually, just like other hospitals. No rational basis exists for distinguishing how these 'public' hospitals are protected.

However, Florida has waived sovereign immunity in favor of defendant substitution. In torts committed by state entities, namely the hospital and nursing home, Florida's waiver of sovereign immunity allows plaintiffs to recover damages from the state government but places a cap on payment of a judgment or claim up to a maximum of $200,000 per person. Our case falls under the 2019 Florida Statutes, Title XLV Torts, chapter 768 Negligence: Section 768.28, which describes the waiver of sovereign immunity in tort actions, recovery limits, and limitation on attorney fees.

The biggest drawback to finding an attorney is that: "No attorney may charge, demand, receive or collect, for services rendered, fees above 25% of any judgment or settlement." By limiting the maximum fee, an attorney can collect to 25%; the legislature reduces the number of cases brought against the state. It is difficult for a plaintiff to find an attorney to work under these limitations. The limits leave plaintiffs with meritorious claims without representation because an attorney can collect up to 40% contingency fees for lawsuits not involving the state.

A firm will spend as much time, money, and effort to represent a client with a million-dollar case and a possible $400,000 contingency fee as it will representing a plaintiff suing the state where the maximum award is $200,000, with a slim chance of getting that sum, with a total $50,000 contingency fee. In addition, as I have experienced, the hospital attorneys, who are on a hefty hourly retainer, intend to take up as much of the plaintiff's attorney's time as possible by slow-walking the case to a conclusion.

Under sovereign immunity, the hospital could, in an operation, remove the right kidney instead of the failing left one. The patient suffers years of pain, has enormous medical bills, and dies of kidney failure. Despite the hospital being guilty of medical malpractice, its maximum liability for this malpractice is $200,000.

In its pure form, sovereign immunity confers absolute immunity from legal liability upon the sovereign, leaving injured parties without any course or compensation. In medical malpractice under negligence law, sovereign immunity and the related concept of defendant substitution can provide significant protection against liability for physicians working on behalf of a state or federal government.

Medicine is a complex endeavor, and the Florida approach is another instructive example of understanding how modern sovereign immunity affects medical malpractice negligence law. While Florida has chosen, for policy reasons, to allow its local governments to be substituted as defendants in medical negligence lawsuits, thereby allowing plaintiffs to recover damages from the state government, the state has also imposed monetary caps on such damages.

Sovereign Immunity details why firms were not flocking to represent me in my case against the hospital and nursing home.

Florida's medical malpractice laws do not benefit patients; they help insurance companies, hospitals, and doctors. The laws in Florida make it exceedingly difficult to pursue a medical malpractice case. It is expensive, and the maximum fee an attorney can collect, based on getting the full damage settlement of $200,000, is $50,000. This return depends on being awarded the top award allowed under sovereign immunity, and the chances of getting the maximum award are slim to none due to court-ordered mediation.

It now becomes the obligation of the attorney to determine whether taking the case is economically feasible. Sovereign immunity is under attack, and academic opinion has been overwhelmingly hostile. It has not served as a bar to effective relief for lawless conduct by state agencies but has operated to defeat claims arising from their actions. In fact, for some time, a substantial number of Supreme Court justices, usually not less than four, have stood poised to end the doctrine.

My search for an attorney to represent us expanded to all Florida firms listed as malpractice law firms. After many rejections and waiting for a response to my case description, I finally got a hit. I received a call from a firm we call LGF in Tampa. After a fifteen-minute discussion with the managing partner, he decided LGF would take the cases. On 5 September, I received the following letter welcoming me and several forms to be signed and returned.

Thank you for selecting our firm to represent you about your potential medical malpractice claim. A file has started, and we request some or all of your medical records. We will review the medical records and other relevant information you provide us. If we determine you may have a meritorious claim, your documents are given to one or more medical experts for review.

After the records review, our experts will advise us on whether we can obtain a declaration of facts supporting the claim. Communication is essential to your case, and we will happily answer any questions you may have, so please e-mail them to us. (*Remember this statement.*) Please remember that medical malpractice cases are lengthy, expensive, and time-consuming. Your cooperation will be one factor in deciding whether to pursue your claim.

I returned my signed documents to LGF to sign and return a copy for my files. LGF still needs to return the signed documents as required by law despite my numerous requests for them to do so. The contract will be detailed later when I receive my copies.

I will briefly detail the contingency agreement. Despite the Florida Constitution limits of a 25% maximum for contingency fees, lawyers who represent clients in medical malpractice cases may charge a price more than the constitution's fee limit with the client's consent. LGF informed me of their intention to set a 40% contingency, and they may petition the court for approval of the fees which exceed the limitations of Rule 4.4-1.5.

To get representation in a sovereign immunity lawsuit, I had no option but to agree to the 40% contingency and sign the agreement. I later discovered that my contract was not legal because the law states that my consent form must be notarized. The Rules of Profession Conduct require that a lawyer who charges a contingency fee in a medical liability case provide the client with a copy of the constitution's fee limitations, a copy of which I did not receive.

Florida Statute 768.28 states that Florida attorneys for claims against state agencies are limited to a contingency fee of 25%. The statute questions the 40% contingency fee agreed to in the contract with LGF. The Court would unlikely rule that the legislature's ability to limit attorney's fees payable out of a claims bill award is unconstitutional because such power impacts access to the courts. Contingency fee arrangements are 'the poor man's key to the courthouse' and guarantee every citizen's right to access our courts.

Subsection 768.28 (8), which puts a cap or 'ceiling' on contingency fee contract compensation, has been held by the Florida Supreme Court as a constitutionally permissible limit on attorney's fees. The right to contract for legal services is a fundamental constitutional right implicating strict scrutiny and cannot be imparted by subsequent legislation which tries to restrict that contractual right. Will my signing a contract agreeing to a 40% contingency fee bind me to that, or does the legislature's mandate that claims against state agencies cannot exceed 25% nullify that contract?

The goal of litigation for medical negligence is to compensate the plaintiff injured by the negligence, discourage the negligence practice, and extract corrective justice. Only 15% of medical malpractice cases have oversight, and information from claim trend analysis from malpractice insurers shows that less than 1% of all filed medical malpractice cases end up in a verdict for the plaintiff. In most cases, the attorney and administrative costs consume the award. Litigation is expensive and inefficient.

In an appeal, a descending judge described the 25% attorney contingency fee as 'draconian' and said it unconstitutionally impairs the contract between attorney and client. Limiting contingency fees for attorneys could restrict court access for many people who otherwise could not afford legal representation. However, the Florida Supreme Court has held that limitations of attorney's fees are a constitutionally permissible exercise of legislature authority and do not constitute an impairment of contractual obligations.

Sovereign immunity is often referred to in this story and applies to the lawsuit where detailed. LMHS is one of the hospital systems in Florida falling under the statutes. Following is the answer provided by the defendant in response to the question, "Describe all policies which you contend cover you for the allegations outlined in Plaintiff's Complaint."

LMHS and HPCC is a public health care system created by a special act of the Florida legislature, Chapter 63–1552, Laws of Florida Special Acts. LMNS is an independent special district under the laws of Florida. As a governmental unit, LMHS, its employees, agents, and related entities are entitled to the Florida Waiver of Sovereign Immunity Act, section 768.28, and the liability limitations.

Chapter 9
Lawsuit Investigation

LGF will start collecting information to substantiate a lawsuit by requesting the hospital medical records and x-rays applicable to Beth's ER visit. LGF will concentrate on their medical experts reviewing the x-rays to see if they can detect the same anomaly her surgeon did. LGF said I should e-mail any questions or additional information. On 2 January, I sent the following information to my attorney.

One of the severe after-effects of my wife's broken tibia, caused directly or indirectly by HPCC, is her susceptibility to urinary tract infections (UTIs). They will occur due to HPCC's actions upon her arrival at the facility. After breaking her tibia, she was placed in a leg immobilizer, making it difficult to go to the bathroom without a CA aid. To eliminate the need for the CAs assistance, HPCC embedded a catheter for her to urinate.

After a few weeks, she complained of having the urge to urinate despite having a catheter implanted. We visited her urologist to see what he could prescribe to control her problem. His first question was why she was on a catheter, not in diapers. He emphasized that the longer she had the catheter embedded, the more susceptible she would be to frequent UTIs. I informed him that HPCC had embedded the catheter without explaining why.

The urologist said he knew why they placed it; it was for HPCC's CA's convenience, so they would not have to take the time to take her to the bathroom or to change her diaper. Thus, a procedure instituted by HPCC for their convenience may result in Beth's being subject to frequent UTIs for the rest of her life.

The warning from her urologist has proven factual. She has had five UTIs since leaving HPCC, all needing hospital stays. Based on a review of Beth's medical records, do we have a meritorious claim or not?

On 1 March, I sent the following; still waiting for the promised case progress reports.

Per your 5 September letter, 'We feel that communication is vital to your case' and 'we are happy to answer any question you may have.'

My past questions must have made you unhappy since I have yet to receive a case update as requested. Getting no response, I logged onto the Florida law website to see my options to get case updates. Their response was to send requests for information by 'certified mail' receipt requested. On 4 May, I sent the first of other certified mail requests.

Numerous requests for case updates have received the response, "You will get back to me with answers to my questions." Refer to your latest e-mail of 13 April, saying I would get an update next week.

"It has been three weeks since the next week with no answers, and I am requesting answers to the following question. Your 5 September 2017 introduction stated that LGF had started a file to begin your preliminary review of the subject medical malpractice cases. Referring to the 'Statement of Client's Rights,' you, the client, have the right to ask your lawyer at reasonable intervals how the case is progressing and to have these questions answered to the best of your lawyer's ability." Inquiry, how are the Medical Malpractice cases going?

LGF answered that our expert is currently reviewing your medical malpractice case. Please give our firm and our expert time to thoroughly review all aspects of your potential medical malpractice case so we can provide the best representation possible. The nursing home malpractice case goes into another phase called NOI or Notice of Intent to put the Defendants on notice. When sent, we will notify you. Our office will contact you when our expert finishes his review and sends us a report about your medical malpractice case.

An NOI definition is a letter establishing a legal issue with someone and giving them notice that you intend to file suit. It tells the other party you are giving up trying to settle the case and will let the Court decide instead. You do not have to threaten a court suit for it to qualify as a notice of intent to file a lawsuit. The NOI states: Please be advised that according to Chapter 400, Florida Statutes, Elizabeth believes you are a prospective defendant in a case involving violating her resident's rights and negligence.

Elizabeth intends to file a lawsuit against you and any others with a legal relationship with you for her resident's rights and failure regarding the care and treatment received. At the same time, she was a resident at HPCC from 18 May 2017 to 29 July 2017. There is a lot more legalization, but one crucial statement is: Per Florida Statute, the parties must meet in pre-suit mediation to discuss the issues of liability and damages. I will cover the mediation procedures later.

In a call on 8 March, I was told LGF is still reviewing the case and that my attorney will keep me updated. I suggested that rather than e-mailing, we schedule a monthly progress conference call to check the case progress. She agreed. After talking to her for the first time, six months into the case, I wanted to be more impressed with her knowledge.

A review of her credentials on LGF's website informs me that she is called a Litigation Associate with a BA in Political Science. She later earned a law degree with experience representing lenders in the foreclosures industry. Not an impressive background to have her representing me in a medical malpractice case. A follow-up e-mail informed me that the defendant got the NOL on 16 April.

I received a letter from LGF on 31 May regarding my nursing home claim. Please find the attached Pre-Suit Interrogatories and Pre-Suit Request for Production directed to you, which you are required, by law, to answer. Interrogatories are questions that must be answered under oath and which can be used in Court.

Please fill in your suggested answers on the enclosed working copies. Try to be as specific as possible on all your questions and answers. The finalized answers to the interrogatories must be filed with the Court within thirty days of the date listed on the certificate of service, so I request that you return your draft answers promptly.

Interrogatories: These are questions submitted by the defendant and must be answered by the plaintiff. The defendant may submit up to thirty questions to be answered by a statement that must be at least one sentence long. The law states that the plaintiff and defendant should exchange information about the facts of the underlying incident, the plaintiff's allegations, and the defendant's potential response to those allegations.

To meet the prompt request, I immediately started the process. There were 23 questions, most of which requested information they already had and others that would not affect the case. By law, the opposing counsel has the right to ask the following questions, and it is my responsibility to answer them regardless of their relevance. Collecting the records would take over thirty days for the plaintiff to answer these questions with all the requested information. These questions, and many like them, will be used by the plaintiff and defendant's attorney throughout the litigation.

A list of the names, addresses, and specialties of all hospitals, physicians, and other healthcare providers, including dental and psychiatric care, visited during the last five years with a brief statement about the treatment rendered by each. Copies of all medical, dental, psychiatric, and hospital records in your possession for the past three years. Elizabeth held positions with the names and addresses of all employers for the past five years. Copies of Elizabeth's tax returns for the past five years.

The educational background of Elizabeth with a list of schools attended during the past five years. Please provide the current names and ages of Elizabeth's children and the addresses of the children at the time of the alleged incident. Give a full description, including inclusive dates, of each injury and illness of Elizabeth during the past ten years. The name and address of the physicians Elizabeth consulted concerning her health condition, specifying the purpose the physician was consulted.

What is the name and address of each hospital where Elizabeth was a patient, setting the inclusive date of hospitalization on each occasion? Other than the alleged incident, has Elizabeth ever filed a lawsuit or presented a claim against any person, firm, or corporation seeking money, damages, or compensation? (To this question, I answered yes that I had filed a lawsuit in 2001 claiming medical malpractice against the parent company of HPCC, the subject of this suit.) Itemize medical and hospital expenses incurred or paid by Elizabeth, the date such expenses were incurred, the name and address of the person to whom each of such costs was paid or incurred, and the dates of payments.

Please state the name and address of each person known or believed by you, your attorney, or other representatives to be: A. an eye witness to the occurrence described in the Pre-suit Notice, and state his location at such time; B. not an eye witness, but or may know the facts upon which the allegations of negligence contained in the Pre-suit Notice are based and state their location; C., not an eye witness, but who has or may have knowledge of the facts upon which the allegations of damage contained in the Pre-suit Notice are based.

These questions were answered briefly while still meeting the answer requirements. I answered the following question in detail. What you are to read has already been stated to other questions and will probably be asked again in the future. Therefore, I will give a capsulized version of my detailed answer.

Q: Describe each act or omission of the defendant you contend constituted negligence contributing to the legal cause of the incident.

A: The embedding of a catheter as a convivence to eliminate the aides having to change her diaper or help her to the bathroom, leaving it embedded far beyond the duration mandated by Medicare guidelines, thus exposing Elizabeth to frequent urinary tract infections. Severe dehydration necessitated Elizabeth to be rushed to the emergency room in a non-responsive state, needing accelerated rehydration to bring her back to consciousness. HPCC knew of her dry condition but did not have a nurse who could insert an IV.

My response to the Pre-Suit Interrogatories was sent to LGF on 4 June to review my suggested answers. I requested a review based on research that states the court allows a party to consult with their attorney when answering interrogatories so that counsel may help their client carefully construct the responses. This collaborative effort can help minimize any damaging effects of the client's responses.

On 15 June, I e-mailed LGF. Not having heard from you, I assume the interrogatory answers I submitted are acceptable, and you need no other information from me. Confirm this belief. No response. On 27 June, I e-mailed once again. Having received no comments on my pre-suit interrogatories, have you submitted my answers to opposing counsel as written? Received no response.

Fed up with the lack of response to questions asked by e-mail, on 10 July, I once again reverted to sending the following certified mail letter to LGF.

I find it difficult to understand that a firm that states, "We feel that communication is essential to your case," is reluctant to do so.

I refer to two recent e-mails which have yet to be acknowledged or answered, a task that a simple e-mail reply could have done. Instead, I must again revert to the Florida Bar recommendation that firms that do not answer requests for information submitted through normal means, the same information be requested by 'certified mail.'

I ask the answers to the following questions on my nursing home claim. Were my suggested Pre-Suit Interrogatories submitted to opposing counsel as written, and, if so, when were they summited? When does opposing counsel have to respond to the Pre-Suit interrogatories?

On 6 August, having not heard back about my 'certified letter' information request, I e-mailed the managing partner. When it becomes necessary for a client to request case information by 'certified mail' because answers cannot be gotten when asked through normal channels, I must assume the system is broken. LGF received the last certified mail request for information on 11 July, and as of this date, I am still waiting for a response.

Based on the above e-mail, I got a call scheduling a conference call with my attorney for 7 August. I compiled a list of questions, hoping her verbal answers would satisfy my inquiries. Not surprisingly, her answers did not; the following sums up our conversation.

Question: Were my suggested Pre-suit interrogatories submitted to opposing counsel as written? Answer: Yes Question: Is it prudent to review them with me before sending them since they were designated suggested draft answers? Response: The answers looked good and will be submitted without modification. Question: When were they submitted? Answer: The answers still need to be submitted to opposing counsel.

Question: Why? You told me on 31 May to return my answers as soon as possible because they had to be submitted to opposing counsel by 30 June. I sent my responses to you on 4 June. You are telling me that as of 7 August, you still need to submit them. Answer: I was out of town but will get them out tomorrow. The rest of the call went downhill from there. I requested we hold a monthly telephone conference so I could ask my questions directly and hopefully get an answer.

I got an e-mail from the managing partner asking if I got my questions answered. I responded that I got to discuss my questions with her on Tuesday, 7 August, but I wanted better answers. For example, on 3 June, I sent expedited answers to the Pre-Suit interrogatories to be sent to opposing counsel to meet a 30-day deadline.

However, on 7 August, 65 days after sending my responses, she told me she still needed to submit the interrogatory's answers to opposing counsel. I do not know when she would have presented them if I had not called. I requested my attorney hold a monthly case update phone conversation. I suggest you institute such a practice.

I will mention this in our next scheduled attorney meeting. Thanks for your feedback. Trust me, it helps.

It didn't help because the monthly case progress calls agreed to on 10 October, as of 19 November, have yet to be present. To remedy this, I scheduled a conference call for 20 November. I then sent her a list of questions I would like to discuss.

I called on the 20th only to be told by her secretary that I was off her schedule and she was on the phone. I repeated that I had confirmed I would call and asked if it was necessary to change that date to e-mail me. I informed the operator to tell my attorney I had set aside the time and date for our call and have her call me when she got off the phone and before four o'clock. Not getting the requested call back, I gave her another opportunity to answer my questions by e-mail with a Wednesday deadline. Still not hearing from her, it was time for me to take corrective action.

On 26 November, I e-mailed the managing firm partner and told him it was time to end my relationship with my attorney. We have no client/attorney rapport, and I no longer have confidence in her work. I detailed the above-missed call information and told him that, in a past lawsuit, I have never had my attorney not give me at least monthly case progress updates. I requested my association with my attorney end and my case assigned to another firm attorney. He responded that my case had been assigned to another attorney. I now start over with my second attorney.

He informed me that the opposing counsel had received the interrogatory's answers, and the next step was to go to mediation. These answers only apply to the nursing home lawsuit, and I will discuss the mediation process later.

Chapter 10
Wife's Deterioration

Beth came home from her rehab at FMR at the end of August when her Medicare coverage expired. She still had the urge to urinate and could not walk without a walker. Most of her day is spent in bed with daily debilitating nausea, which starts first thing in the morning and lasts most of the day. She can navigate from A to B, but B has become the bathroom, and she makes multi-trips to it hourly.

Her daily mantra continues to be "I got to pee." When she tries to do so, little or no urine comes out. The pain must be excruciating, but no correcting medication can alleviate the feeling. The only web-listed remedy was exercise, which she could not do, and pelvic exercises. As for nausea, she underwent many tests, and the medical professionals could find no physical explanation for her sickness.

She started physical therapy three days a week at home. The workouts went well, but several had to be canceled because of her nausea. She is still very unsteady on her feet, and in November, during one of Florida's hurricanes, she fell. Getting EMTs to transport her to the hospital was impossible because of the weather conditions.

The next day EMS took her to the ER, where she was again diagnosed with a severe UTI. The culture grew a bacterium the hospital could not identify this time, and they consulted CDC to determine it. It came back as sepsis, and the only way to treat it was to place a PIC line in her arm and administer the antibiotic intravenously for ten days.

The hospital thought a home nurse could administer the shot daily, which proved impractical. The Infectious Disease Medical Department instructed me to take Beth to the ER so the hospital staff could perform the infusion. To free up a hospital bed, she was sent to a nursing rehab facility where they could complete the daily injection.

Again, let me digress here. After the infectious disease, the doctor told me to return Beth to the hospital. I got a letter from the hospital telling me her admittance was on observation status. I would be liable for 20% of her hospital bills since Medicare does not cover the hospital stays on an observation basis.

I again objected, saying Beth was readmitted to the hospital at the request of the infectious disease physician so a medical procedure could be performed. I stated she was admitted to the hospital on a need basis, not an observation status, and Medicare should cover her stay. It was. Remember the ER case Worker telling me the hospital would not admit Beth on an observation basis?

On 10 November 2017, she was admitted to the WC rehab facility so the nursing staff could administer the daily anti-biotic. The medication cost was $1192 for the ten days, which I had to pay because the medication was not on our prescription drug plan formulary. A rule of thumb is that every day spent in bed equals losing three days of physical therapy. She started occupational and physical therapy twice daily to compensate for the lost ten days needed for the infusion.

The room charge of $254 per day for the 21 days she was in the facility was covered by Medicare since she had spent the required three nights in the hospital, making her eligible. However, the $875 physical therapy costs were self-pay because she had used all her Medicare physical therapy allotment at HPCC. In early December, she was discharged and came home to continue in-home physical therapy.

She continued to suffer daily nausea, which limited the days she could do physical therapy. Starting in March 2020, she had occupational or physical therapy seven times at home. Wanting to get her out of the house, I rescheduled her treatment with a physical therapy unit found in a PT facility. She received another twenty-two days of occupational and physical therapy, but it did not significantly improve her walking ability. After the last sessions, they told us the condition she was now in would be as far as she would progress, so there was no reason to continue her therapy.

Hearing this diagnosis just accelerated her depressed state of mind. She did not get outside except for her Thursday hair appointment and our trip to Perkins for dinner. The odd thing was that her nausea usually ran from early morning until around three o'clock, and whenever she went to the hospital with severe nausea, they could never duplicate it while she was a patient. She would leave the hospital feeling OK but down with a sickness the next day.

She had undergone a brain scan, several endoscopies, blood work, and even had her gall bladder removed but could find no physical cause to explain her constant nausea. We even tried four one-hour hypnosis sessions to see if that would help alleviate nausea. Being a licensed hypnotherapist, she enjoyed the sessions, but the sessions did nothing to relieve her nausea.

I researched the web to match her symptoms with a cause and found a condition that matched her symptoms. I suspected her nausea was psychosomatic. It is previously described as a somatic symptom disorder, where a person feels nausea despite no physical cause. Since nausea could not be duplicated in the hospital, I suspected it might be an environmental cause since nausea returned when she returned.

To prove or disprove my belief there might be a home environment connection, her many trips to the bathroom increased her possibility of falling when I was not home; I entertained the idea of getting her out of the house. To confirm my belief that the nausea was a bodily condition and to ensure that if she fell, there would be a helping attendant to call, I placed her in an assisted living facility for a thirty-day trial.

Surprisingly, the change reduced her daily nausea; thus, a change in environment confirmed my SSD diagnosis. As a side, her gastroenterologist agreed I had made a diagnosis the medical profession has been unable to solve. He even took the case to a symposium of gastroenterologists in Baltimore.

However, the urge to pee did not go away, and she became a disruptive facility resident because she constantly called for a CVA to take her to the bathroom. The continual calling became a situation that could prevent her from becoming a resident on a full-time basis. She returned home after the thirty days stay, nausea returned, and the trips to the bathroom were as frequent as ever. I then decided my only solution was for her to return to the assisted living facility full-time.

Having long-term care insurance, I expected no trouble getting approval for Beth to go into assisted living. I was wrong. I knew there was a ninety-day elimination period before long-term care kicked in. Still, it was evident that her hundred days in rehab under Medicare met her ninety-day elimination period since the days covered by Medicare count as elimination period days.

When the long-term care policyholder asked for proof of completing the ninety days, I sent them Medicare's statement showing she had used all her 100 days and was no longer eligible to draw Medicare for the year. The insurance company informed me that the Medicare document was unacceptable and that they needed itemized monthly billing from each rehab facility. The information request required all the rehab facilities she had been in to compile a list of her stay costs detailing her room, her medications, the facility's license, and a copy of the current Minimum Data Set Assessment. The MDS is a document the nursing home must complete at least every three months.

The facilities sent in the documents they thought the insurance company wanted but were told the forms needed to be more specific and to submit corrected copies. The facilities told me this was nothing new because the insurance company was a pain in the ass to deal with. Eventually, the company received all the needed documents and approved her stay.

Before determining whether the facility met the insurance companies' requirements, the assisted living facility had to prepare a whole new set of documents showing their nursing facility meeting all the insurance company requirements, plus sending in a current MDS.

In addition to the facility-needed documents, Beth had to be evaluated by an insurance company nurse to see if she met the requirement of being unable to perform two of the six activities of daily living. (Bathing, Continence, Dressing, Eating, Toileting, Transferring) She met that requirement, the facility gave all the necessary documents, and she was approved to pay monthly assisted living costs.

The facility took her back because I would pay an extra fee for CAs making trips to her room to quiet her down when she called for them to take her to the bathroom. Her room cost was $3360 per month with the added price of $375 for medication dispensing, $221 to help her to the dining room, and $265 for additional care for a monthly total of $4314. I also furnished the room with a bed, dresser, chair, and table for $2400. Her long-term care insurance covered her room and services costs.

She adapted well to her new home, spending time watching television and working continuously on 'word unscramble' puzzles. We played Scrabble several times weekly, and she had no trouble making words and adding points. I made it a point to join her every night for dinner. However, she was becoming more disruptive, screaming for help to pee, going out into the hall looking for me, and showing more dementia-related symptoms.

At the end of August 2018, I visited Beth at the assisted living facility. It was raining, so I started to run for cover upon exiting the car. Then it happened. I heard my knee pop, accompanied by shooting pain, and could limp to Beth's room. I sat and told her what had happened; she thought it might be a pulled muscle. When I tried to stand up to leave, I could not and called for an aide to bring me a wheelchair and call EMS to take me to the hospital.

After three hours in the emergency room and taking x-rays, the doctor told me nothing was broken and to see my orthopedic doctor the next day. I was issued crutches and now had to try and get a cab at 12:30 AM to take me the five miles back to my car at the nursing home. I managed to get the car and got home at about 1:00 AM. The next day, I saw my orthopedic doctor, and he suspected it was a torn meniscus.

An MRI confirmed his belief, and surgery is scheduled for 6 September. I underwent arthroscopy knee surgery, relying on my neighbor to take me to and bring me home from the surgery center. He remained on call as I went through the pain associated with wearing off the anesthesia. Two days later, I started my eight weeks of rehab. Since it was my left knee for the eight weeks, I could drive and make my daily trip to see Beth.

The medical problem the urologist told us would become more frequent due to the extended embedding of the catheter was her coming down with urinary tract infections (UTIs). From her August assisted living facility admission through December, she came down with three UTIs, two of which required her to be admitted to the hospital for a three and four-day stay.

Each set her condition back, and she became weaker after every hospital visit. Her mobility decreased, and she never seemed able to recover from each visit. One of the significant symptoms of a UTI is confusion and memory loss, and it became more noticeable after each visit that her short-term memory diminished.

In November, I started noticing a change in Beth's behavior. When she entered the facility, she would spend hours doing word Scrabble puzzles, but now she complains of constant pain, and all she wants to do is sleep. I am also getting reports from her neighbor and the staff that she is starting to leave her room and roam the halls calling for me. Her neighbor had my phone number, and anytime she was being unruly, he would call me, and I, ten minutes away, would rush over to the home and calm her down.

It is now becoming evident that she is in early-onset Alzheimer's and would eventually have to move into the memory care unit. In February 2019, a room became available, and the move was made. Her condition had worsened, not her memory, but she had become weaker, complained about constant pain, and wanted to sleep all day. Another coincidence is that her last nursing job was in this same memory care unit, where she was the charge nurse for twenty-five Alzheimer's patients. The room and service cost for the memory care unit went to $6413 per month.

She adapted to her new room and returned to watching television and doing her word puzzles. We even once again played a few games of Scrabble. She could also navigate with her walker to the bathroom whenever the urge to urinate and no longer needed to call the CA to take her. She could dress, change her ileostomy and walk to and from the dining room for meals.

She adapted well for a month, and then she became noticeably weaker and weaker. Her memory faded, and her ability to walk diminished. It became readily apparent that she was sick, and I decided to have her taken to the emergency room. Once again, she was diagnosed with a severe UTI and admitted.

Between November and April, the hospitals in town are running at 120% of capacity. The time of year when the 'snowbirds,' the visiting northerners, are in town and have no local doctor, use the emergency room as their doctor's office. All the emergency rooms are full, patients are on every gurney in the halls, and people are sitting in chairs waiting to be seen by a doctor.

She was taken to the hospital in an ambulance; she got an ER room and spent the night there awaiting a bed in the hospital. She remained in the hospital with intravenous antibiotics and intravenously administered magnesium because her magnesium was low. Her other blood work was not standard, but they did not treat blood deficiencies, and she was returned to the facility.

When she returned, she was in the best shape she had been in for months. Even the staff commented that she was more alert and had more energy than they had seen since she came to memory care. Physical therapy was to start the following week. However, her condition deteriorated two days after getting back from the hospital. She progressively began to become confused and was losing her ability to walk.

The therapy was started, but she was too weak to take part. She could no longer stand or walk and became dependent on the CAs or me to get her to the bathroom and dressed. I told the nursing staff I thought she still might have her UTI and asked them to take a urinate sample and have it tested. The first test returned negative, and I was at a loss as to why her condition had deteriorated rapidly.

On April 10th, I put her to bed, and she was almost non-responsive. I debated my next move when I got a phone call at 11:00 PM telling me Beth had fallen and sustained a large bump on her head. They wanted my permission to send her to the emergency room, which I gave them.

Once again, the hospital ER was packed, and her transport by ambulance got her a bed in a room because they needed the equipment to diagnose her condition. She once again had a severe UTI. Her doctor told her that it appears the doctor anti-biotic prescribed for her UTI two weeks ago was not the right one to treat a UTI this serious.

She had a mastectomy on the left breast, and the nurse should not take blood work from that arm. To make matters worse, as described by nurses, she has tiny veins, and it is almost impossible for them to get blood. Usually, the nurse must call an intravenous specialist to get a line in to draw blood. Her UTI and other blood work results needed her to be admitted to the hospital as soon as a bed became available. So once again, she spent the night in the emergency room.

She would not return to the memory care unit, so I informed them she would leave. I had one day to get all the furniture out of the room since the items belonged to me and the unit did not want them. Her room rent would continue if there were furniture in the room, so I spent the day transporting the furniture in the back of my SUV to store in my garage.

Her UTI was bad, and she had other problems resulting from many past UTIs. Upon admittance to the hospital, she had third-stage kidney failure, which increased to the fourth stage at discharge. She also cannot maintain an acceptable magnesium count, possibly due to her kidneys filtering out the mag. The UTI was the major problem being treated, and one has the constant urge to urinate with the infection.

Since it is a problem, the condition makes the desire more substantial and consistent. The continuous crying that she had to pee necessitated her moving from a two-person room to a single room closer to the nurse's station so they could get to her quicker. She continued trying to get out of bed to go to the bathroom, a trip she was not to make, so the hospital put a sitter in her room to prevent her from doing so.

The search began to find a skilled nursing facility with an open bed for her. Rehab beds are scarce, and we contacted several facilities to see who had availability. She will now fall under Medicare for the first 20 days of her rehab and Medicare plus her secondary insurance for the next 80 days, thus covering the costs of her stay.

The hospital noted in her medical reports that she would go to a skilled nursing facility upon discharge. Thus, she could not return to her memory care room because they were not a skilled nursing facility and had already occupied her space with another resident. It now became the responsibility of Beth's Case Worker to identify skilled nursing facilities that had a bed open in their memory care unit.

She found two, WC and MC, who could take her. She mentioned that MC had a representative in the hospital I could talk to about sending her there. This representative might be like a lobbyist who roams the hospital halls to see who is being released and needs a rehab facility. I should note that MC was a for-profit facility while WC was not, so I suspect the representative may be getting a commission from the facility for patients sent to them by her.

I reviewed the facility to determine its suitability for Beth's care. It was not an impressive building, needing a parking lot resurfacing and increased landscaping. However, it was unique, with a large bird enclosure holding six tropical birds in a comfortable lobby. I talked to the Admissions Director and explained my situation, and she informed me that since her doctor in the hospital was also MC's doctor, he was aware of her condition. After a tour, I was impressed with the facility and agreed to her be sent there for rehab.

On April 25th, Beth was transported from the hospital to MC and given a bed in the memory care unit because of her continued crying out, "I have to pee."

She was the only person in the two person-bedroom. I initially wanted her to get out of the room to eat in the dining room, but after seeing the condition of many people in memory care, I thought the dining room was too depressing, so I had her meals delivered to her room. I found meals to be my most significant dissatisfaction with the facility.

I usually visited for a few hours at noon and evening. I found the lunch meal delivered to the room at 1:30 and dinner at 7:00, typically cold. I have accepted that she would have to live with this situation.

She was evaluated and started occupational and physical therapy two days after arrival. I found the therapist to be very professional, but Beth was a pain in the ass. All she wanted to do was sleep, and when they came to get her for OT and PT, she said she could not do them because she was too sick. Failure to do PT defeats the purpose of rehab, and if she continues to refuse the therapy, they would report she was not making progress, and Medicare would no longer cover her stay.

Medicare covers the first eight days at the total cost, at which time her progress is evaluated, and if progress is reported, Medicare covers 80% of the price. My secondary insurance covers the remaining 20%. If there was no improvement and I needed her to stay, I would pay 100% of her costs.

On April 29th, I received a letter informing me of my daily cost. My 20% share of the cost would be $171 per day, thus making the room's total price $853 per day. MC listed the services covered by Medicare (room and board, therapy, medications, wound care, incontinence products, special nutritional items, trach care, ostomy care, oxygen, special mattresses, x-rays, labs, nursing services, activities, social services, physician visits) with no cost per service shown.

I will not inquire about fees until the first in-service meeting, which details her progress and determines whether her progress meets Medicare's criteria for continued coverage. Whether she met the requirements made no difference since I had no choice but to leave her in the facility at $853 per day while I hunted for somewhere else to take her. The nonprofit WC fees were $254 per day, and PT was another $40 to 50 per day for $304.

To add to the costs, hundreds of dollars of medications still in the prescription bottles used to treat her while in memory care at BD were considered unacceptable by MC and could not be used because all the medicines must come from MC's pharmacy. The same goes for Pampers I supplied being replaced by diapers furnished by MC.

On Thursday, 2 May, I visited Beth at 11:00 PM, just as they were ready to take her to OT. She was in bed and just as weak as she had been lately. The therapist helped her into a wheelchair and took her to rehab while I remained in the room. At 1:00, I started walking down to the rehab area only to meet her and her PT therapist coming up the hall. She was in her wheelchair, and the therapist had her push herself up the aisle by manually turning the chair wheels.

I then took over and pushed her back to her room for lunch. As usual, the aide had already brought lunch to the room, which was cold and unappetizing. Again, she did not eat, drank a little of the Coke I got her, and said she was sick and had to go to bed. I dressed her in her nightgown, put her in bed, and left.

When I returned at 6:00 PM, she was not in her room, and I found her in her wheelchair sitting in the depressing dining hall with an uneaten meal in front of her.

She said, "Get me out of here." I told her I would take her back to the room after eating.

Again, she commented, "I cannot eat this crap; I must lie down." I took her back, dressed her in pajamas, and put her to bed. She complained of being sick and so weak I had to lift her legs into bed. She could not move in bed and asked me to turn her on her side.

I got upset and told her, "You can do it by yourself," but it became apparent she could not. I told her she should be sitting up; all she wanted to do was sleep. I left in a huff thinking she was playing me for sympathy.

When I got home, I felt terrible about my departure and asked myself if maybe she was extremely sick and exhausted. I decided to go on the internet and research fifth-stage kidney failure and found that all her symptoms matched. It then dawned upon me that she was dying. Beth is not saying she is sick to get out of doing physical therapy but because she is sick.

All I could think about was what my next step was. Should hospice be called back for another consult, should I begin hunting for a long-term care bed, and ask MC to take a respite blood workup to confirm my contention that her kidneys were failing and she was dying? I spent a sleepless night staring at the clock, arising at 5:00 AM, and spent the next hour trying to decide her future and my options.

My options are limited. If confirmed that Beth is in kidney failure and not a rehab patient, she will go off Medicare and revert to self-pay at $853 a day until I can get her into a long-term care bed. This search for a bed could last indefinitely. Should I contact hospice and see if a bed is available in their facility?

My last hospice representative said Beth, a past hospice volunteer, may get some priority for admittance. Should I inform MC of my dying belief or wait until the Care Conference on 9 May? I headed to the golf course for a 7:00 tee time with all this on my mind. Again, my playing partners sense something is wrong, but I have not shared my troubles. I have chosen to keep my family troubles to myself.

On 9 May, I was to have my review and planning conference to determine Beth's continued treatment. I have had these meetings in other facilities, and the discussions had the facility administrator and the two therapists giving her occupation and physical therapy. The therapist filled me in on her progress and gave me a projected schedule for her to reach her therapy goals. I could ask questions about her therapy progress and agree to meet again in two to three weeks.

The meeting at MC was utterly different. After waiting an hour, I was joined by the Social Services Director and no others. He then looked at his laptop screen for five minutes, which told him Beth was making progress with no other comments about her goals for the next few weeks. He repeated; that she was making progress. Those two words, 'making progress,' ensure the facility continues to collect its $852 a day for the next 100 days from Medicare and my secondary insurance. Letting Medicare know Beth is making progress ensures that Medicare will continue to pay its daily expenditure.

I asked him to detail the services that went into the $852 daily fee. He said the room costs $325 per day and $100 for physical therapy, and I would have to address the question of the remaining $427 costs with the business manager. He insinuated why I should care about what made up the costs since Medicare and my secondary insurance covered them? I told him I did because if Beth had to remain beyond the 100 days, I would pay the $852.

On 17 June, I toured a recently built care facility with one memory care room. I liked the facility and returned to MC to see when physical therapy expected Beth to use a walker, a condition she must meet to go to the memory care unit. PT projected that she would meet those criteria in two or three weeks. Using that estimate, I paid the $1500 facility down payment and scheduled an occupancy date of 3 June. However, when Beth was rushed back to the hospital, the need for a memory care room became moot.

Chapter 11
Medical Malpractice Case

The hospital malpractice case is less promising than the nursing home case. LGF hoped to make its case on the ER physician not seeing the break on the x-rays and a review of the ER dictation. My first review of the case was when I read the 'Emergency Room Dictation' and proceeded to contradict statements made thereon.

Statement: "XR of left knee reviewed by a radiologist, and I show no fracture and osteopenia. In addition, the Pt complained of pain radiating from the knee down her leg, but no scans or XRs were taken below the knee." I responded that if the patient complained of leg pain, why weren't additional XRs taken?

Statement: "At 7:40 PM, Pt could ambulate in the department." This statement is false, and she was not ambulating, as documented by her inability to walk to the bathroom at discharge.

Statement: "The Pt was informed of her results, and her diagnosis of pelvic contusion" is also false. Our only encounter with the attending physician was his telling us, "Good news, there are no fractures," and he was gone. A recording attendant did not accompany him, so he wrote this statement afterward.

Statement: "Pt is agreeable and verbalizes understanding" is partially true in that I understood what the Case Worker was saying but strongly disagreed with her being discharged. The patient's complaint of pain was responded to by saying, "She has no broken bones, and the pain she is suffering was normal pain experienced with a bad fall."

Statement: "Results were reviewed as displayed above" is false. The only review of the results was the 'good news' statement, and I never got to ask the doctor why, with no broken bones, my wife is complaining of severe pain below the knee.

Statement: "The Pt was given a treatment plan." The caseworker would immediately request Home Health Care to call my wife in the morning, a request never made.

Statement: "At 8:06 PM, Pt was able to emulate with some difficulty," another false statement. The patient was moved, with extreme difficulty, from the bed to a wheelchair because she could not walk without assistance. The nurse recognized the patient's pain and applied an ACE bandage below the knee.

Statement: The final diagnosis was a pelvic contusion, which no longer describes the condition diagnosed on her return to the ER the following day.

Statement: The referral to counseling was 'the pain is normal to fall pain,' and she would contact Home Health to set up a physical therapy schedule. I responded, "How will she do PT when she cannot stand up without pain?" I disagreed with the discharge plan, but she would still be discharged despite my objection.

Statement: The scribe did not personally see the comments made by the physician. The treatment, procedures, and medical decision-making were discussed with the patient; a stock statement was attached to the ER visit. Information should have been discussed with the patient. Never once is the term 'road test' mentioned in the dictation.

Statement: On page 19, for the first time, the report stated that 'Pt needs to be assisted with ambulation.'

The first information I received on the case came in an e-mail sent on 17 July 2018, stating that LGF's expert has reviewed the medical records and believes the radiologist may have missed the fractures on the ER x-rays. He informed LGF that radiologists often overlook this type of fracture (tibia/fibula).

X-rays taken on 12 and 13 May were not sent to our office and have been re-requested by the radiology department. Our expert will review these and make a final determination about your claim. My interpretation of the above is that LGF's expert made his assumption based on reading the records and not the X-rays, which I believe he can only make by seeing the X-rays.

On 10 September, LGF informed me that their medical experts needed help to determine whether the ER doctors had missed seeing the tibia break on the x-rays. Based on my past lawsuit, which I will document for you, I told them we might spend too much time and money trying to prove a subjective position and should be looking at an objective situation. I am not trying to self-lawyer, but the attached narration may be beneficial.

In 2002, Beth accepted a medical malpractice lawsuit settlement from the same hospital corporation. In that case, we did not seek damages from the principal doctor. Instead, we sought damages based on nursing staff negligence, showing they did not follow the standard post-operative hip replacement surgery protocol. Their failure thus resulted in permanent nerve damage to Beth's foot.

Since your medical experts cannot agree that the ER doctors missed a tibia break on the x-ray or that they should have taken an ultrasound of the lower leg, the facts remain that the last shattering of the tibia was not a result of the failure of the doctor to see, but a result of the ER discharge nurse's negligence. The discharge nurse did not perform a valid 'road test' as ordered by the doctor and repeatedly requested by me.

Requests for the nurse to see if my wife could walk to the bathroom without pain were ignored, as was my request to see the doctor, being told the doctor had released her. The nurse did not instruct Beth not to weigh bear on the leg until she saw an orthopedic doctor. The discharge nurse had trouble getting my wife in the car without her complaints of pain, and I asked how I would get her out of the vehicle. The nurse said she should be able to walk the short distance, again not emphasizing she did not weigh bear on the leg.

When I requested the Case Worker admit my wife to the hospital on observation status, she denied the request saying it would be 'too expensive.' When I told her: "you can see my wife is in obvious pain when she tries to walk," I was told, "This is just normal pain associated with a fall." The actions of the nurse and Case Worker were the primary cause of my wife shattering her tibia and having to return to the hospital the next day.

The above-listed negligence of the discharge nurse and Case Worker is cut and dry and does not need expert evaluation. I am sure discharge protocol can be obtained from the hospital and reviewed for compliance.

As for the hospital, saying my wife's return was because of a fall was false. She did not fall but collapsed. A fall is 'to move to a lower position under the effect of gravity,' whereas collapse is 'to fall suddenly, to cave in due to the loss of support,' namely, the tibia shattering when weight is bearing on the leg.

She would have ended up prone on the floor in a fall, but this was not the case. In her attempt to go up the 5" step from the garage to the house, as soon as she put weight on the injured leg, her leg collapsed, and she ended up sitting.

This collapse, rather than a fall, was evident from the ultrasound image taken on her return to the hospital, which showed a total shattering of the tibia and not just a break that would have resulted if it were just a fall. It is readily apparent that a simple fall from a standing position to a prone position would not have caused this much damage to the tibia.

Her ortho doctor informed us the shattered tibia was probably the result of a stable tibia fracture that broke once she placed weight on the leg. He believed she should not have been discharged from the ER without further testing. I would suggest LGF investigate the objective nursing malpractice and not the subjective attempt to show that the doctors should have found the break when they viewed the x-rays.

Medical negligence is defined as "A doctor or hospital is liable for medical malpractice in Florida if the healthcare provider failed to provide reasonable care, skill or treatment of the patient." This can include "a hospital nurse failing to respond to a patient in distress."

I further informed LGF that they established the case file on 5 September 2071, and here it is a year later, and the firm has yet to determine whether there is a malpractice case. LGF stated they are diligently working on the matter and would follow up on my suggestion that the ER discharge protocol is investigated.

On 18 October, I sent the following message to LGF. As a follow-up to my contention that ER discharge protocol is a more promising issue for pursuing a malpractice suit, I submit the next experience. On Monday, the quick care clinic sent me to the ER with what was suspected to be a heart problem. After many tests, they found no cause for my dizziness and unsteady gait.

The doctor said he would discharge me, pending the nurse performing a 'road test.' When.' I failed the test because I still had an unsteady gait, the nurse informed the doctor, and he admitted me to the hospital. I give you this background to support my contention that my wife's ER nurse did not follow proper protocol and should have notified the doctor when she saw my wife could not walk without pain. As an aside, I was suffering from vertigo.

The second episode concerns my request to the Case Worker that she be admitted on observation status since my wife could not walk without pain. Her telling me it was not the hospital practice to admit on an observation basis because it would be too costly to the patient was false. Upon discharge, my Case Worker gave me a 'Medical Outpatient Observation Notice' to sign, "You are a hospital outpatient receiving observation services that require further time and reevaluation to determine the severity of your illness and whether you require hospitalization."

The Case Worker attending my wife's ER visit was incorrect when she said it was not hospital policy to admit on an observation basis. It would be very costly to me if they admitted me on an observation basis was also incorrect. Admission on an observation basis means Medicare will only pay 80% of the cost, and I would have to bear the remaining 20%, which my secondary insurance covered, so I had no out-of-pocket cost.

In addition, I received a GH treatment survey. To question the ER nurse discharge protocol once again, I submit the following questions from the survey:

Before you left the emergency room, did you understand your main health problem? Before you left the emergency room, did you know what symptoms or health problems to look for when you left the emergency room? Before you left the emergency room, did someone tell you to make an appointment with a doctor to follow up on your problem? Before you left the emergency room, did someone ask if you could get this follow-up? During the emergency room visit, did doctors and nurses give you as much information as you wanted about the results of the X-rays?

During the emergency room visit, how often did the nurses explain things in a way you could understand? How often did doctors/nurses listen carefully to you during the emergency room visit? During the emergency room visit, how often did doctors/nurses explain things in a way you could understand? Did the doctors spend enough time with you during the emergency room visit? In my wife's case, the answer would be no to all.

On 31 October 2018, I got a letter from LGF addressing my medical malpractice case.

Thank you for considering our law firm to represent you in a potential medical malpractice claim. I have come to fully appreciate the tremendous personal impact that medical negligence can have on the lives of those whom healthcare providers have improperly treated.

You should be aware that a medical negligence action differs from other types of lawsuits. In suing a doctor or other health care provider for malpractice, the burden is on the injured party to prove by expert testimony that the health care provider deviated from the prevailing standard of care by improperly supplying or not providing proper medical care and treatment.

In addition, the law required testimony from qualified medical experts to show that the departure from the prevailing standard of care directly caused or contributed to the injuries sustained.

The law in Florida requires that to testify as an expert witness in a claim of medical negligence against a health care provider; the expert must have the same or similar background, skills, and training as the potential defendant health care provider.

Our experience is that the medical and legal elements involved in a medical malpractice claim can be proven only after extensive review by qualified medical experts of all the medical data and other documentation related to the case, usually at considerable expense. It is challenging to find doctors to testify against other doctors, and we often find it necessary to consult out-of-state doctors, thus adding to the cost.

Unfortunately, upon review of the medical records, we could not find an expert willing to say that a failure in the applicable standard of care exists. Our emergency room expert reviewed the medical records and said the radiologist should have read the imaging during the 12 May emergency room visit. The CT scans and X-ray taken on 13 May showed an injury not visible in the 12 May imaging.

We consulted an emergency room expert at your suggestion to ask whether the 'road test' discussed applied to the emergency room nursing staff under these facts. While emergency room nurses often conduct a 'road test' for patients with respiratory and breathing issues before discharge, no similar application or mandatory pre-discharge test was administered to patients with ambulatory problems.

(This contradicts my experience of being given a 'road test' to see if I could ambulate without difficulty. The nurse notified the doctor when I could not, and he admitted me to the hospital.)

Instead, she directed us to the 12 May nurse's notes, stating that at 7:25 PM: "Patient was able to pull herself up out of the stretcher and assume a standing position with the walker. The patient could take steps and walk with a walker but complained of pain with each step. The patient's husband states she cannot walk with a walker, and he wants to see the doctor." (As stated, never once does it mention the patient could bear weight on her injured leg. Her ability to ambulate depends on the walker bearing her, so the 'road test' validity is questionable.)

The doctor verified this, saying the patient could ambulate with some difficulty, and discussed mobility/care with case management. (The doctor never returned to see the patient and used the nurse's notes as his only progress report, and he never saw her try to walk. In addition, when discussing mobility care with the Case Worker, why was the patient not informed not to weight bear until she saw her ortho doctor.)

The emergency room nurse later noted at 8:06 PM that the patient's husband wanted her to try to go to the restroom with a walker. The patient stood up with a walker and asked, "Where are we going." I explained that we were going to try and walk to the restroom. The patient states, "I can't; it hurts too much."

Placed ace wrap on patient's left knee where she complained of pain. The patient states, "Make it tight." The patient refused to ambulate with a walker and notified the provider that it was too painful. (The nurse's notes duplicated my description of earlier events. She was discharged despite the patient's complaint of excruciating pain.)

The nursing expert noted that under these facts, the emergency room nurse's responsibility—and the applicable standard of care—was stressed, and notifying the doctor of these ambulatory issues and that in the context of the doctor's diagnosis of a pelvic contusion, there was no reasonable basis for the emergency room nurse to override the doctor's discharge orders.

Rather than blaming the discharging nurse, the malpractice charge provided the nurse gave the correct ambulatory problems information to the doctor should be directed to the doctor for not doing a proper follow-up on the nurse's notification of pain experienced by the patient when trying to ambulate.

The Florida medical association proposed and lobbied for the medical malpractice legislation enacted in Florida. The legislation has increased difficulties for claimants to pursue medical negligence cases within the brief period existing law allows. The burdensome procedural requirement of Florida medical malpractice law has afforded a great deal of protection to doctors and other medical professionals.

It has created significant obstacles for individuals injured or damaged by negligent medical care. In part, these legislative changes have been a factor in determining whether the costs of bringing a medical negligence claim would be justified when weighed against the amount of any potential benefit to the claimant. The statutory limitations on the damages recoverable means that the expense and risk of accepting medical malpractice cases often outweigh the possible compensation if a claim is accepted.

Unfortunately, this means that meritorious medical malpractice cases often cannot be taken on a contingency fee basis. The situation you have related to me has been reviewed considering the abovementioned factors and my experience. Unfortunately, your case does not meet our law firm's criteria for further action. Therefore, we cannot undertake your representation. Our decision not to represent you further is based on several factors, including economic ones. This does not mean that you do not have a right to sue or that this claim does not have merit, but only that this case does not meet our firm's criteria.

Should you want to pursue this matter further, you should immediately contact another attorney. Based on all the information above, I accept LGF's decision not to pursue this claim further. The case may have merit, but the expense of following it far outweighs the monetary benefits if the issue is decided in our favor.

Chapter 12
First Mediation

Mediation allows two people having a dispute to talk about their issues and concerns and make decisions about the conflict with the help of a mediator. A mediator cannot decide who is right or wrong or tell you how to resolve your dispute. In medication, you can find solutions that make sense to you and the other person in the conflict to resolve some or all of your concerns.

Now, why were we at mediation? The defendant had three options after receiving the claim. First, the defendant could reject the lawsuit, which they had not done, or we would not be here. I can conclude that the defendant recognizes that the incidents described in the Pre-Suit interrogatories are factual and did occur.

Option two was that the defendant could make a settlement offer. Again, I can conclude that the defendant did not exercise this option because the plaintiff may have accepted a settlement offer, thus eliminating the need for mediation. Option three is that the defendant can offer to mediate in which liability is admitted. The defendant took option three.

Mediation benefits only the defendant. In this case, the defendant has a maximum liability of $200,000 due to sovereign immunity. Thus, the defendant's sole purpose of mediation is to reduce that liability payout, so the plaintiff cannot get the maximum liability short of going to arbitration.

For the privilege of going to mandated mediation, the plaintiff faces a reduction in any damage award and incurs added legal and mediation fees. Even though the defendant admits fault and must pay damages, they plan to mediate them as low as possible.

The mediator's background shows his experience emphasizing personal injury matters and his familiarity with nursing home disputes. Since he cannot give input on the case, his experience means nothing. The definition of mediator function is to make those in conflict come to a fair agreement.

What criteria does he use to decide what a fair deal is? With no medical background or enough knowledge to determine the severity of the defendant's negligence, how can he determine what is a fair agreement?

Mediation was held on 20 March 2019 in Ft Myers. By my having Beth's 'power of attorney,'' it would not be necessary for her to be at mediation. I met my counsel, who had driven down from Tampa for the first time.

In the discussion, I learned my attorney came out of a family law practice he and his wife had, and he was bored with family law and thought injury law would be more enjoyable. I questioned how an attorney with a family law background could litigate a complex sovereign immunity lawsuit.

The mediator introduced himself and said his only duty was to convey settlement offers between the parties. He would have no opinions concerning the case but would only be the messenger between the two parties. His fee was an estimated $600 per hour with a three-hour minimum.

The mediation expenses were to be shared equally between the two parties. Even though we are in mediation because the defendant did not exercise option one or two described above, the plaintiff is still responsible for footing half the expenses.

Opposing counsel entered the room with a registered nurse specialist from the hospital. Their counsel read from a written report which, to sum up, said the nursing home was not responsible for the incidents described in the complaint because the facility followed the advice of the doctor, who was not an employee but a sub-contractor.

I stated that I had a contract with the facility and expected them to furnish Beth with competent medical care. I saw that the incidents described in the suit resulted from nursing and staff incompetence, not doctor incompetence.

Mediation figures are confidential, so the numbers used are hypothetical. The process description is not privileged because it can be found on many websites. We made a settlement offer of $200,000, the maximum cap under sovereign immunity.

Opposing counsel said they would take it under advisement and adjourned to another room. The mediator went with them to get their response to our offer. After about fifteen minutes, the mediator returned with a counteroffer of

$1,000. We reduced our settlement offer to $165,000, which they countered with $3,000.

The mediator informed us that the defendant's parent company would not settle for a six-figure offer. We then said fine and reduced our settlement offer to $95,000 to see if they intended to resolve this matter in mediation. Again, the mediator took our offer next door and returned with a counter of $7,000. It was at this point that I decided mediation was over. I was willing to end the mediation session and would file for binding arbitration.

The mediator was paid approximately $1,800 for the two hours he spent walking between rooms, and all I got out of it was his expenses plus the expenses of my counsel to make the trip from Tamp. It became apparent that the opposing counsel had no intention of settling the case in mediation. Florida law requires parties to a lawsuit to attend court-ordered mediation in good faith. The defendant did not follow the good faith mediation principle and was there only because the court mandated it.

This farce concluded the mediation step in the lawsuit process. According to my counsel, the next step was to prepare the documents necessary to inform opposing counsel that we intended to go to Voluntary Binding Arbitration.

Arbitration is if there is reasonable preliminary ground for a medical negligence claim after the pre-suit investigation is completed, either party may request an arbitration panel rather than a court to determine damages. (As per my attorney, the parties must go to arbitration and not trial by contract.) If the opposing party accepts, the acceptance is a binding commitment to comply with the arbitration panel's decision, provided no settlement is reached beforehand.

My attorney said he would start the process immediately by requesting arbitration and keep me informed. With mediation ending on 20 March, I enquired on 11 and 18 April whether my attorney notified opposing counsel of our intent to go to arbitration, receiving. Getting no response, I got fed up with my attorney's lack of action and entertained the possibility of firing my attorney and seeking new counsel. I called the law firm I had initially submitted my case to see if they might be interested in taking over the matter.

I talked with an attorney who explained the difficulty of firing an attorney. It involves dividing any settlement funds as to who is entitled to what percentage. Finding an attorney to take over the case would be difficult, especially in a sovereign immunity case. Facing the difficulty of changing my attorney, I decided to stay with what I had.

On 26 April, I reverted to using certified mail to inquire whether my attorney had started the process of serving a request to opposing counsel for voluntary arbitration. When a client must revert to requesting case update information by 'certified mail' because requests made by e-mail go unanswered, I must assume the attorney has such a heavy caseload that he cannot take the time to answer a yes or no question.

It may benefit the client and the attorney to remedy this situation by seeking representation elsewhere. My leaving would reduce the attorney's caseload by one client and allow him more time to answer other clients' quests for information—your call.

On 2 May, I called my attorney, getting his secretary, who inquired about the purpose of the call. I told her I wanted to know if the opposing counsel had obtained the documents necessary for binding arbitration. She said they had.

The notice of wanting to go to arbitration is not just a letter saying so in the legal system. Like all legal proceedings, you cannot simply do anything. The Summons is a 19-page document sent to the nursing home and their parent hospital. It must be served on the defendants by the sheriff and states as follows: YOU ARE COMMANDED to serve this Summons and a copy of the Complaint in the above-styled cause upon the defendant: (HPCC and LMHS).

Said Defendant is required to serve written defenses to the said Complaint on Plaintiff's Attorney within 20 days after service of this Summons and to file the original of these written defenses with the Clerk of this Court before service on Plaintiff's Attorney immediately after that. If the defendant does not do so, a default will be entered against that defendant for the relief demanded in the Complaint. On 29 April 2019, the summons was registered with the court.

There are 15 pages headed up COMPLAINT AND DEMAND FOR JURY TRIAL. COMES NOW, through undersigned counsel, Plaintiff ELIZABETH files this complaint against the defendant and alleges GENERAL ALLEGATIONS, listing 36 allegations of noncompliance and negligence. In addition, the nursing home's Summons request DEFENDANT SHALL PRODUCE THE FOLLOWING ITEMS AND MATTERS and then describe 64 items and matters.

At the defendant's response time expiration, I e-mailed my attorney to ask if opposing counsel had responded to the summons. On 20 May, receiving no response to my e-mail, I called the Clerk of Courts directly. Since the defense counsel had to file a response with the court, I asked if the court had received that response. The Clerk told me they had no record that the summons had been served on the defendants contradicting the secretary who told me it had.

I immediately called LGF, got the same secretary, and asked why the summons was not served. She thought the Sheriff had served them.

I said, "What do you mean you thought they were served?"

"Didn't you get a notice from the sheriff when they had been served?" she said she would get on it, see if they were served, and call me back. Getting no callback, I called the Court Clerk, who informed me the summons was served on 22 May. The warrant issued to the defendant means nothing unless the sheriff serves the defendant's summons. I could not understand why a law firm would prepare a 54-page subpoena, submit it to the court on 29 April and not serve until 22 May.

On 12 June, the defendants responded to the summons by filing a MOTION TO DISMISS and MOTION FOR MORE DEFINITE STATEMENT AND MOTION TO STRIKE. The filing of this motion to dismiss is standard procedure by defendants.

The plaintiff starts a lawsuit by filing a complaint with the Clerk of Court and serving a copy on the defendant the summons. Instead of answering the complaint by admitting or denying its allegations, the defendant responds by filing a Motion to Dismiss (MTD). The MTD is supported by a defendant's claim that a complaint is inadequate or improper.

In our case, the defendant says, "Now moves this court to enter an order dismissing Plaintiff's Complaint, and enter an order requiring Plaintiff to plead with more specificity and enter an order striking a portion of Plaintiff's Complaint as follows." The defense lists 14 items the defendant considers vague and needs more specificity, another way the defendant slows down the suit's progress. The plaintiff must answer the motion.

"'Defeating the motion to dismiss is critical because your entire lawsuit can be thrown out of court if you lose.' Therefore, your written response to the MTD will be critical."

Not getting a copy of the defendant's written defense submitted on 12 June, I paid a $7.00 copy charge and purchased a copy of the MTD. It listed 14 items the defendant was disputing, which I chose to answer myself.

On 5 July, I e-mailed my attorney asking if he had prepared an opposition memorandum to the MTD. I have answered all the defendant's 14 points as specified in his motion. No response. On 7 July, I e-mailed again, asking him the time frame specified by the court to file a response to the MTD. No response. On 19 July, my attorney sent me an e-mail asking me to send him my answers to the MTD. It appears I was to be the one to prepare the answers.

However, on 8 July 2019, addressing this MTD was no longer relevant because of the plaintiff's death.

Chapter 13
The Ending

On Tuesday, 11 June, I got a call from MC informing me Beth was in a fib, had shallow blood pressure, and was sent to the ER. Arriving at the ER, I found the waiting room full and the emergency room hallway filled with people on gurneys and chairs, but Beth had a room. The first urinalysis showed she once again had a UT, but more troubling was that GFR kidney function was 13.9, with a count below 15.0 being fifth-stage kidney failure, and her creatine level was 3.33, with 1.06 being the top of the range.

These results signify that her kidneys are not functioning, and she will be admitted to the hospital. However, a problem usually unheard of this time of year is the hospital being at 120% of bed capacity. She would have to spend Tuesday night in the ER and hoped a bed would be available tomorrow.

A bed became available in the hospital Wednesday evening, and she moved to a room. Once again, she complained about having to pee even though bladder scans showed the bladder to be empty. The hospital put her on a new type of catheter that fits outside her and works by suction, developed to end embedded catheter problems.

The hospital is now treating the UTI with antibiotics and intravenous feeding her fluids to get the kidneys to function. She receives the solution for the next five days, and blood work is taken twice daily. Treatment got the kidney function up to 32.0, but the kidney function will diminish once again when treatment ends. One good happening was that our son, who lives in London, was in town and got to visit her. Little did he know this would be the last time he would see his mother alive.

She screams, "I got to pee," driving the nursing staff up a wall daily. Tranquilizers and anti-psychotic medications have not been adequate to end the problem of feeling like she must pee all the time. She is also not eating, and her mental and physical condition is deteriorating.

On Friday, 13 June, I had a hospice consult to see if she was a candidate for hospice care. Their representative determined she met the criteria for hospice admittance since she is in end-stage Alzheimer's and will experience kidney failure soon. I signed the papers on Saturday approving her move to the hospice house.

A hospice bed problem delayed the move until Tuesday, 18 June, when a bed in the house became available. As in the hospital, she started her "I have got to pee" mantra as soon as she was in the hospice bed. Hospice put her on an embedded catheter, not ending her crying out. Telling her to pee because she had a catheter did not relieve her feeling. By experimenting with different depression medications, they could finally calm her cries but not end them.

Hospice will discontinue many prescribed drugs and only treat her with mood-stabilizing and pain medications.

As hospice states, "Hospice care is designed to meet a resident's physical, emotional, and spiritual needs. You acknowledge that hospice care is focused on providing comfort, pain relief, and symptom management."

She now sleeps most of the day and is not eating.

She is dying. Saturday, for the first time, she ran a fever of 101, which is a sign of infection.

She is not eating or drinking little, her breathing is raspy, and she keeps repeating, "God, please make me better" or "I have got to pee".

The catheter remains, but there is little urine in the bag, a sign of kidney failure, and she could have another UTI. We will not know because hospice does not do blood workups. Their function is to keep one comfortable and out of pain. I make two trips to visit each day, and enduring her suffering is getting harder and harder.

I suspected Beth again had a severe UTI. Although I know hospice will not treat the infection, I did ask the nurse, for my information, to take a urine sample and have it tested for a UTI.

On 25 June, I met with the social worker at the hospice to discuss Beth's future stay at the house.

The RN informed me they had stabilized her, and she was not yelling, "I got to pee," and "God, please help me get better" continuously. Still, it will take another week to determine whether she will remain in a hospice house or move to a continuing care facility.

Beth keeps telling me, as she has many times, "I am sorry to put you through all this suffering, and it is all my fault." Her apology was heartbreaking, and I assured her I did not mind spending time with her.

Her condition continues to decline. 2 July was the first time she did not recognize me when I visited. Her kidney function is starting to fail, and the nurse informed me that she is in the process of dying. It is getting harder and harder to watch her daily decline.

Today, 3 July, I went to visit after golf and got to talk to the PA. She informed me that they are changing her medication to calm her down again. She told me she would be sleeping more when I visited.

They are trying to control that when she wakes up, she automatically screams, "Nurse" or "God, please help me."

These outbursts are what they are trying to control or eliminate. Beth does not know she is screaming and cannot stop the impulse to do so. The PA told me her urine output is decreasing, which may signify her kidneys are failing. Hospice tries to measure the resident's time to live, and Beth is in the days to weeks category.

Through all this, my day goes like this. It starts at midnight when I go to bed, and if not asleep in half an hour, I get up and read till two o'clock. I am up at 5:00, getting my usual four to five hours of sleep a night. Read the paper, have a healthy breakfast, and be on the golf course by 7:00. I play daily.

On Sunday, I go out the back nine by myself. Golf is my quiet time, where I have the course to myself and think about Beth's upcoming death. I have not told any golfers that Beth is in a terminal condition. I am very private about her situation and don't want the daily 'How is your wife doing?" I have prepared and loaded her obituary into the e-mail, ready to be sent. When the time comes, they will all be notified immediately.

My 4 July visit found Beth repeating 'nurse' repeatedly, and she no longer recognizes me. The PA told me the results of a brain scan taken in April showed swelling of the cerebral cortex, probably the source of her repeating the exact words repeatedly. The medical staff has been trying to stop this screaming with different medications for the last few weeks.

However, this brain scan shows no prescription will correct this condition, and the nurses will block all attempts. I will reduce my daily visits from twice to once a day since she no longer knows whether I am there. We are now on a death watch.

On a 5 July visit, I found Beth awake with her eyes wide open but not seeing. Her every breath is accompanied by a groan continuously until she falls asleep. Her mantra has gone from "nurse" to "God, please make me better," along with the now-present groan. The nursing staff has learned to recognize this and no longer answers her cries since they can do nothing.

I have decided to reduce my two times a day three-hour visits to a one-time fifteen-minute visit. She no longer knows if I am there, and my looking directly into her eyes and addressing her gets no response. She no longer eats and is getting liquids only by a mouth swab.

The nurse told me it takes fourteen days of not eating to die and ten days without drinking. She is dying, but the process is slow, and eventually, her kidneys will fail and shut down her vital organs, concluding the death process. It is now just a matter of time.

Today, I asked the administrator if hospice could use her wheelchair, walker, crutches, and portable toilet, and they gladly said they would welcome my donating them. They would use all of the items in the hospice community of patients having home hospice services. Donating these items recognizes that Beth will never again use them and would be of more excellent value to others who need them.

Hospice notified me that Medicare payments for her stay in hospice had ended, and her remaining would now be subject to private pay. Paying is no problem because Beth has long-term care insurance covering the $175 per day charge. It makes one wonder how those who need skilled nursing services can find the money to continue these services. It becomes evident that dying can become expensive, which could place a heavy monetary burden on a substantial number of caregivers.

I learned firsthand of a caregiver who moved from his northern home to Florida to tend to his mother. He had sold his house and belongings to obtain the funds necessary to make a move and now has no possessions left to sell to continue the payments required to keep his mother in a long-term care facility. It now becomes evident that death is more expensive than living.

For example, Beth's rehab facility would have charged her $15,392 monthly for a skilled semi-private room or $16,247 for a private room before coming to the hospice. I realize this is a for-profit facility, but moving into such a facility may be necessary to get the help your loved one needs with bed shortages. Many people do not realize the value of long-term care insurance until they are too old to get a policy. For many, living in old age is not always a blessing if it brings the health problems that may go with it.

After my volunteer duties in the library on Saturday, I visited Beth. Upon entering the room, I noticed that the nursing staff had covered her with a new warm blanket, knowing she was always cold; I knew this was a gesture she appreciated even though she could not tell them. Also, as usual, the channel on the television was playing 'Easy Listening' music loud enough for her to hear. She was lying on her back with her mouth and eyes open, and her breathing labored but no longer groaning with each breath.

When awake, she would repeat, "Please, God, make me well," not knowing that even God could not help her now. I bent down to kiss her, but she was not seeing despite her eyes being open. I sat with her for an hour, holding and squeezing her hand but getting no response.

For the first time in her presence, I shed tears of sorrow. I told her I loved her, and she tried to speak, but no words came. I left when she closed her eyes, hoping I would soon get the call that she had passed away.

On Sunday, I got an e-mail telling me there were new test results on Beth's My Chart page, a website showing all the latest test results 24 hours after being taken. The urine culture results showed a 100,000 CFU/ml growth for enterococcus faecalis A and Candida tropical A; in other words, she has a severe urinary tract infection.

Hospice will not treat the condition, eventually shutting down her kidney function. Today, she showed more significant congestion in her lungs, but she continues to hold on to life. In the evening, I got a call telling me Beth's breathing had gotten shallower, so I rushed over to spend some time with her. After a half-hour with her, she seemed to breathe better, so I left.

I got the call I expected at 5:30 Monday, 8 July 2019. Beth died at about 5:15. The last three years of pain and suffering ended. When I got there, I went into room 18. The lights were on, and Beth was in bed with a rose-colored blanket covering her shoulders. Even in death, the staff remembered her always being cold, and she would have appreciated this gesture. I held her hand, which was still warm, talked to her for fifteen minutes, kissed her forehead, and went to the nurse's station.

They had her rings in a bag, and I signed for them. The only other item she had was her favorite foam pillow which I said I would take. I signed the form for the cremation service to take the body. I went in for the last time, held her hand for a minute, kissed her again, and left. She died twenty-four days before our sixtieth wedding anniversary and thirty-nine days before her eighty-fourth birthday. Sixty years of togetherness ended as I walked out the door.

I had e-mailed one of my golfing friends, telling him I would not be at golf today and would e-mail him later to explain why.

My not playing golf would have pissed Beth off because she told me, "I never want you to miss a round of golf because of me."

I had preloaded her obituary into an e-mail and sent it to all the recipients. The next step was to call the newspaper and inquire about getting her obituary into tomorrow's paper. I can see where the newspaper's obituary section is a profit center. The obituary cost $394.30, and a picture was another $30. I spent the next hour figuring out how to take a picture of an image, load the photo disc into the computer, and e-mail it to the newspaper.

I got help from the computer tech support, the camera tech support, and the girl at the newspaper before successfully transmitter her picture. I then called social security, the prescription drug plan, and the insurance company to report Beth's death and make changes. My next task was to meet with the cremation society to sign the necessary papers and place the following obituary in the paper.

Elizabeth was freed from pain when she died in Hope Hospice on 8 July. Born Elizabeth (birth name) in Akron, OH, on 15 August 1936, the family moved to DuBois, PA. After graduating from high school in DuBois, Beth graduated from the nursing program at Columbia Hospital in Pittsburgh and started her professional nursing career in the operating room.

She worked as an emergency room, industrial, school, and geriatrics nurse, licensed to practice as a registered nurse in five states. Beth was also a Certified Hypnotherapist, getting her certification in 1998. She finished her working career at the Lakes Nursing Home in Ft Myers.

She and her husband moved to Ft Myers from Buffalo, NY, in 2000, where she volunteered for Hope Hospice and the Friend of the Library and joined the Catholic Community. She is survived by her husband of 60 years and her son John Alan living in Dubai, UAE. The US Navy Burial at Sea Program will conduct a memorial service before her and her husband's ashes when he passes.

The rest of the evening was spent reading the replies to the e-mails. It was also the first day of my changing routine. For the last three years, every day at noon and 5:00, I would visit Beth in the hospital, rehab, assisted living, memory care, and finally, hospice. I always tried to get there at lunch and dinner to eat or feed her. I will miss the daily trips.

On Tuesday, my computer crashed and was out of service for the entire day, making it impossible to answer the people sending me messages about Beth. I also had my appointment with the cremation society to sign sixteen forms for death certificates, agreements for the cremation, and other documents required for the service.

I was expecting to pick up her ashes but was informed that cremation would not be done for up to fifteen days so the medical examiner and the doctor could sign off on a cause of death. I will not be able to bring her home for two more weeks.

As for the cause of death, my diagnosis is that her numerous UTIs in the last years resulted in kidney failure, which shut down her vital organs. I contribute it to the defendant's embedding of a catheter against all medical advice that catheters not be inserted unless medically necessary and removed as soon as possible. The catheter remaining embedded for over seventy days was the major contributing cause of her frequent severe UTIs.

I look forward to making the defendant pay for their malpractice. My problem is that my WebMD does not qualify me to make a diagnosis.

On Wednesday, I started golfing again, not looking forward to the 'Sorry about your loss,' surprisingly, it was not too bad, and I had no qualms about accepting their condolences. Also, I solved the computer problems, and my life started returning to normal. On Thursday, 11 July, I sent the following e-mail to my attorney reporting her death.

Elizabeth passed away on Monday, 8 July, in hospice. The contributing cause of death, as confirmed by a hospital urine analysis, was a severe urinary tract infection (UTI), which shut down her kidneys. The UTI and the many others suffered before this one directly resulted from HPCC's embedding of a catheter.

They're leaving it in for an extended period, despite Medicare's mandate to nursing homes that 'a catheter will not be inserted unless medically necessary and removed as soon as possible. To quote the CDC, "UTIs are the most common type of healthcare-associated infections and are most often caused by the placement or presence of a catheter in the urinary tract." To quote further, "'repeated UTIs' will lead to kidney failure."

The weekend has arrived; it is time to remove Beth's belongings. The first to go is her fine collection of beautiful clothing. It is hard to imagine they will all be hung on racks at the Salvation Army store. Her diamond ring will be shipped to New York to be sold at auction, and her hearing aid will go to a donation center in Minnesota. Next is to dispose of hundreds of dollars of medications and supplements. Now what to do with her collectibles, teapot collection, Mickey Mouse figurine, and basket collection?

When Beth bought them, she thought her son would like to have them when she passed, but times have changed, and items she thought would be valuable to her son have now become clutter that he has no interest in taking. He is collecting valuables for his children, who will consider them clutter when the time comes.

When I pass, my son should sell the house furnished, and I recommend these items go with the place and become someone else's problem to get rid of when they depart. This experience impresses the importance of cleaning up my estate so my son will not have to go through this same disposal task.

On Tuesday, 23 July, I traveled to the cremation society office to pick up Beth's ashes and the death certificates. Per her mandate, I never miss a golf day because of her; I played nine holes before picking her up. Eighty-two years of living and sixty years of marriage are now in a 5" x7" x9" white corrugated box containing her ashes.

The package was surprisingly heavier than I thought it would be. The cremation society placed the parcel in a blue shopping bag for me to carry her out. The bag is nice, but it has the cremation society's name on it, so I do not think it would be a bag you place on a grocery store checkout counter. I placed the load on the front seat and put on the seat belt for the last time for the trip home, the home she had longed to return to for the previous three years.

I attached a picture to the box and placed it in a place of honor in the living room. She will remain there until my passing when my son will put us both in a container and ship us to Jacksonville, Florida, US Naval base. We will be taken out on a naval vessel and buried at sea.

Today is 1 August, the date we got married sixty years ago. I had the same anniversary card I gave her every year, just changing the year. Now I am trying to figure out what to do with the card. This was the day we hooked a trailer to a 1956 Buick her father gave us and started our marriage by driving to Alabama. Who could even imagine what events would occur from this day? She fell twenty-four days short of getting that card again with the number sixty written inside.

Two weeks after our anniversary was her 15 August birthday, when she would have been eighty-three. This date in 1989 was when she spied a giant stuffed dog in the window of a toy store in Montgomery and fell in love with it. So naturally, I bought it for her birthday, and the dog has traveled with us to all our destinations for the last sixty years.

It sat in our bedroom when she was home and moved with her to the assisted living facility during her stay there. It is now my task to bag it and donate it to the Salvation Army to see if they can give it to some child who can extend his life, not knowing they are getting a sixty-year-old dog. The dog's passing is the last of Beth's memories leaving the house.

Chapter 14
Wrongful Death Lawsuit

Readers may find this hard to believe, but the death of Beth now swings a promising medical malpractice case for the plaintiff to a slam dunk case for the defendant. The attorneys know they could settle this with Beth's death in months, but the defendant's retainer fee attorney will draw it out for years.

In mid-July, I got a strange text message from my attorney sent from his phone rather than by e-mail. He complained that he did not like the way I asked questions and said he went to law school and did not expect to be treated this way, and my questions are more demanding than requests—my response.

A request for information is a request whether the request has a 'please' prefix or not. We both have Law Degrees, so you know, "The attorney works for the client, and the client works with the attorney." You may know more about the law, but I know more about the case, and my knowledge and presentation in arbitration, if the case ever gets there, could be a significant factor in determining your paycheck. Keep me updated on the case progress, and I will not swamp you with questions.

However, I do have one. Did you get the death notice I sent you? It has been five days since I sent the death notice, and I have not heard any word from our counsel. The apparent action on the part of the attorney would be to call the client's spouse and bring him up to date on the next steps or at least express his condolences. He has spent over two years on her case and does not acknowledge her passing. I am slowly setting up an adversarial relationship with my second attorney.

I received an e-mail from my attorney asking, "Are you planning on hiring an estate lawyer" I answered, "No, because she had a will and I was the executor, so why would I need an estate lawyer." His following e-mail states, "I must hire an estate lawyer to proceed with the claim," I answered. Not to be critical, but why did you not send the second e-mail before the first? You do not ask me whether I have hired an estate attorney but should tell me I must hire one.

You are supposed to be my legal advisor. In addition to the above, why didn't you call or e-mail to inform me that the case went from medical malpractice to a wrongful death suit as soon as you knew of Elizabeth's death? Does this mean the present lawsuit has ended, and the case must start again?

On Monday, 22 June, I called my attorney or the managing director and was told they were out of the office. I requested that either return my call today when they returned. My call was to set up a conference call to get several questions answered, which needed to be answered when requested by e-mail.

On Tuesday, receiving no callback, I e-mailed, threatening to file a complaint with the Florida Bar, saying I cannot get case information when requested by e-mail, not get phone calls returned, and revert to certified mail to get information responses. I also sent a list of questions I wanted answered. I also inquired whether they were confident they could handle my case. The last question pissed them off, and they let me know that LCF was dropping my case.

Their e-mail also said, "In response to your threat, please seek new counsel." It further said, "You are free to do whatever you feel is best for you; he also suggested setting a telephone conference with your lawyer next time so he can answer all your questions instead of threatening the attorney. Threats break down the trust factor essential to the attorney-client relationship." I responded.

Before detailing my e-mail, let me say it is not easy for an attorney to withdraw from a case that is in litigation. It is infrequent for an attorney to submit a Motion to Withdraw from a lawsuit. While a client can fire a lawyer at any time, for any or no reason, the inverse is not valid. Lawyers are expected to see each matter through to its conclusion. The Law Governing Lawyers shows that even where cause exists, a lawyer may still not withdraw if he believes the harm caused by the withdrawal will be disproportionately more significant than the harm to the client if the representation continues.

However, the client's consent must be informed, meaning the client has been advised and fully understands the consequences of the lawyer's withdrawal. The client should be allowed to refuse permission to withdraw. An attorney must give the client adequate notice of his intention to withdraw and explain the implications for the client. Lawyers should document the conversations and consultations with the client about withdrawal.

Failure to obtain the required permission and protect the client's interests could pose a potential liability for malpractice and disciplinary sanctions to an abandoned client. An e-mail informing me that a Motion to Withdraw has been filed with the court does not meet the procedure described above for informing the client. I went to the court and obtained a copy of the Motion to Withdraw filed on 2 July 2019.

COMES NOW counsel for the Plaintiff, Elizabeth, and herby files this Motion to Withdraw from the representation of the plaintiff, and like reasons, therefore, states as follows: The attorney-client agreement between the parties has deteriorated, to the extent, that counsel for the plaintiff is no longer able to represent the plaintiff effectively. (My answer is that they have yet to represent me effectively since receiving the MTD on 12 June. Nor have they communicated with me since that date.)

Plaintiff and counsel for the plaintiff must speak about the progress of the litigation more effectively. An impasse has been reached as to the attorney-client relationship. Counsel can no longer effectively represent the plaintiff due to this fundamental communication breakdown in the attorney-client relationship. (They must mention that only the attorney has broken down the communication channel.)

They certify that a true and correct copy of the preceding was given to Elizabeth on 2 July 2019. Once again, this is not true. The only notice I received was the notation on the bottom of the e-mail telling me a motion had been filed, and I had to go to the Clerk of Court and buy a copy of the Motion to Withdraw that I was supposed to receive from my attorney. I welcome their withdrawal, but finding another attorney to take over a litigation case is a significant problem. I will describe this problem later—in my response to the e-mail.

Yesterday, I called you and was told you were out. I specifically told the operator to have you call me back on Monday, the day of my call. The call's purpose was to set up a conference call, as you suggested in your last e-mail. You do not return calls or answer e-mails; I must revert to certified mail to get answers. It is only reasonable to expect a client's attorney to call the new plaintiff immediately after learning of your client's death.

In two years, I have had one telephone conversation with you. In a prior communication, the managing partner promised you would make monthly progress calls, a commitment never kept. If it takes threats to get you to respond, then so be it. Before formally filing the Florida Bar complaint, I gave you a 'heads-up.' I can work with you, but I expect you to perform your obligation to keep me current on case progress.

For example, after our mediation on 3/20/19, you said you would get right on starting the procedure to begin voluntary arbitration, and you filed the same on 4/23/19. Serving the summons going with the arbitration filing was, according to your secretary, served on the defendants. However, when I asked you for their required response, my requests were ignored again. Calling the Clerk of Court, I learned the summon was served on 5/21/19.

An MTD was filed by opposing counsel on 6/12/19 and has yet to be answered as of 7/23/19. The promised monthly calls would have brought me up to date on this matter without my having to threaten you to get them discussed. I am not firing you, but that is your call if you insist on leaving. I am willing to talk to you before you exit if desired.

I called my attorney after receiving the above e-mail and spelled out why I made the threat. I referred to item 9 on the 'Statement of Client's Rights'; you, the client, have the right to ask your lawyer at responsible intervals how the case is progressing and to have these questions answered to the best of your lawyer's ability.

Having a law degree, I ask more questions about legal procedures than your average client but humor me. I reminded him that it is pretty complicated to petition the court to drop a client near the end of a suit. He agreed with my comments and gave me answers to the eleven questions I asked, and decided he should have kept me more up-to-date. He said the firm would review its decision to drop me as a client.

The next day, I was informed that after a review of yesterday's conversation, my attorney agreed to do a better job of keeping me informed, and the firm would keep me as a client. I do not feel good about threatening a formal complaint against the firm, but my pissing them off got the results I have been looking for, and hopefully, we are back to a good attorney/client relationship. He also informed me that LGF had filed a motion to rescind the Motion to Withdraw filed with the court.

It would have been interesting if this matter had gone before a judge, where the attorney would have had to justify their withdrawal motion. The law states there are specific reasons an attorney can withdraw from a case, especially an issue that had proceeded to the point it had, and a client seeking case update information is not one of them.

After hearing my complaints and my objection to the firm withdrawing, it is doubtful that the court would have granted the motion to withdraw. We had a court date to discuss this motion, but the attorney's move to rescind the action canceled the hearing. Questions I asked.

Q: Did you answer the MTD?

A: No. A response may not be proper. As attorneys, we strategically take specific actions to help our clients. There is no time frame to respond to an MTD because the defendant's counsel must get on the judge's calendar for him to hear the motion and make a ruling thereon.

Q: After receiving word of your client's death, why didn't you call to update me on the next steps?

A: I asked if you were hiring an estate lawyer because you must open an estate if any distributions from the lawsuit were made.

Q: Have you filed the client's death with the court?

A: A suggestion of death should be filed after you are amended as the estate's representative. You will then become the plaintiff.

Q: Does this case now become a wrongful death case?

A: Potentially. I do not understand this answer because attorneys have told me the wrongful death case is added as a new claim. I am waiting for clarification from my attorney. As an add-on to the above e-mail, my attorney noted that I am sorry for the loss of your wife. It has been fourteen days since I told him of Beth's death; this is the first acknowledgment.

A formal estate must be opened in all Florida wrongful death lawsuits. The reason being a dead person has no standing to bring a claim. A formal estate is a legal entity formed to house the assets, and usually, the estate's primary asset is the settlement proceeds from the case. I will be named Beth's representative. The estate is the source that brings the wrongful death suit to the court with a court-appointed personal representative, me, in this case, who has the power to prosecute the case on behalf of the estate.

Any time a person's death 'is caused by the wrongful act or negligence' of another person or company, Florida law requires the case to be brought as a wrongful death case. Nursing home negligence in Beth's case fits this criterion. A wrongful death claim is a civil lawsuit in which a family member sues another person or company to hold them accountable for their negligence that caused the family member's death.

Florida statute states that a wrongful death cause of action must be based on conduct that amounts to a wrongful act, negligence default, or breach of contract. The conduct upon which the cause of action is based must have caused the death, and such behavior must have entitled the person injured to keep an action and recover damages if death had not been ensured.

Two examples of wrongful death are applicable in this case: When a physician or mid-level provider prescribes and embeds a catheter without a medical necessity, as described by CMS20068, and disregards the consequences of doing so, and this conduct was a contributing cause of death. A wrongful death claim is brought against HPCC nursing home for providing services that fall below the standard of care expected from the facility.

I contend HPCC was guilty of the above-listed negligence, with justification for that contention being HPCC'S knowingly violating CMS 20068, as previously detailed, in their embedding of a 'urinary catheter' with no clinical condition demonstrating that catheterization was necessary. In addition, HPCC violated all the other mandates on catheter use described in the directive.

I contend there was no reason, other than for the convenience of the facility, that Beth should have had a catheter inserted. The facility should have been aware of Medicare's directive that a catheter not be inserted unless medically necessary. They should also have been aware that violating the Medicare mandate would subject the resident to urinary tract infections. Those infections would increase the longer the catheter was left inserted.

As described previously, Beth did incur many UTIs severe enough to be hospitalized. Physicians recognize that frequent UTIs will eventually result in kidney failure. A hospital urinalysis was taken before her death, showing Beth had a serious UTI, which contributed to her kidney and vital organ failure.

Again, after receiving my bill for $700 for hospice, the long-term care insurance company balked at paying it. They required a current MDS, which hospice is not required to file, and my informing them of this did not satisfy the insurance company. They needed a letter from hospice telling them what I had just told them. The company also wanted a Medication Administration Record or a medication list if the MAR was unavailable.

Once again, I told the company that hospice care is focused on providing comfort, pain relief, and symptom management, so the record of medications or the history of medicines would be meaningless. They did not accept my explanation and wanted a MAR. Finally, the hospice sent a letter saying they did not have to complete an MDS and listed the medications given to Beth. Even though they received an itemized bill and all the other documentation they requested, the insurance company would need fifteen working days to review the claim.

I paid them $1600 a year for the last twenty years for Beth's insurance, and it takes them over a month to approve a $700 bill. Despite the trouble getting approval and payment, the insurance was worth the cost. For the assisted living facility and the hospice cost, the long-term care payments amounted to $40,800. The total premiums for the last twenty years amounted to around $29,000, so the insurance was worth the cost. Making a $1,600 annual premium was much easier than paying the reimbursed $40,800 out of pocket.

Our original lawsuit sought damages under the Survival Statute, which was applicable when the claim was for medical negligence; however, the claim for damages fell under the Wrongful Death Statute upon Elizabeth's death. Following is a history describing why this is necessary.

Under prior statutory provisions, a plaintiff could bring two separate and independent causes of action for a negligently caused death and pain and suffering. At one time, a plaintiff could claim damages under two different statutes simultaneously.

The ability to file two claims was based on the Florida legislature amending the survival statute to read, "No action for personal injuries and no other action shall die with the person, and all actions shall survive and maybe instituted, maintained, prosecuted and defended in the name of the Personal Representative of the deceased."

Under the original provisions of Sec 200.023, along with Florida survival and wrongful death statutes, in a scenario where a nursing home violated a resident's rights, and they later died due to unrelated causes, the decedent's estate would have had a continuing Chapter 400 remedy for the wrongful conduct under the survival statute and a wrongful death action.

In 1973 the legislature restructured the system, enacting the Florida Wrongful Death Act. This act merged the survival action for personal injuries which cause death and the wrongful death action into one proceeding only when the illegal conduct caused the death. It eliminated all claims for the pain and suffering of the decedent from the time of injury to the time of death.

Thus, when a personal injury to the decedent results in their death, no action for personal injury shall survive, and any such action pending at the time of death shall abate. This suit is brought under Florida Statute 400.023, which states, "Any resident whose rights are specified in this part are deprived or infringed upon shall have a cause of action against any licensee responsible for the violation. This action may be brought by the Personal Representative of the deceased resident's estate when the cause of death resulted from the deprivation or infringement of the decedent's rights."

The suit initially sought damages under the Survival Statute when the case was medical malpractice litigation. The lawsuit became a wrongful death action seeking damages under the Wrongful Death Act upon Elizabeth's death. The damage caps are the same for both measures.

In merging the two previous steps, the legislature transferred the items of damages, the decedent's claim for pain and suffering from the date of injury to the date of death, to the new statute. Substituted, therefore, was a claim for pain and suffering of the decedent to the survivor, with the explicit purpose being that any recovery should be for the living and not the dead.

A 1975 Supreme Court of Florida opinion on wrongful death action said, "When a personal injury to the decedent results in their death, no action for personal injury shall survive, and any action pending at the time of death shall abate. The primary difference is to merge the steps and transfer pain and suffering damages from the decedent to the survivors. The legislature intended that a separate lawsuit for death resulting from personal injuries cannot be a survival action but in a consolidated form under the Wrongful Death Act."

"Under the old act, it allowed a separate survival action for the pain and suffering of a decedent. The result would be to enable claims both for the pain and suffering of the decedent under the survival act and for the pain and suffering of the survivors under the Wrongful Death Act. This result would allow multiple actions and claims for pain and suffering contrary to the legislature's clear intention. The court held that the Wrongful Death Act effectively combines the steps and transfers pain and suffering claims from the decedent to the survivor."

A descending vote stated that the statutory language within Section 400.023 conflicts with Section 46.021 of the Florida Statutes, which provides that "No cause of action dies with the person and all causes of action survive."

Chapter 15
Arbitration Prep

Voluntary binding arbitration is another statutory alternative dispute resolution process that parties to a claim may use to resolve their differences. Any party to the noticed lawsuit may offer to submit to the pursuit of voluntary binding arbitration (PVBA) to resolve their case without litigation. The defendant admits liability, and the arbitration process is to determine the claimant's damages.

Arbitrations have a three-person panel. Under the Wrongful Death Act, the law sets parameters for the allowable damages awarded by the panel in a sovereign immunity case at a maximum of $200,000. Florida's statutes allow the plaintiff to recover judgments more than the sovereign immunity cap if the state legislature authorizes it in an official act. It would take years for the legislature to approve the extra amount.

I don't believe this case will go to arbitration, but I cannot assume the claim will not go to PVBA. Since the damages awarded by the arbitrators may depend on my presentation documenting the medical malpractice incidents, I prepared the following description of each.

You have previously read much of this production, but it is new to the arbitration panel. I must show that non-medical catheter insertion and non-responsive dehydration contributed to Beth's death. Explaining events substantiating our medical malpractice claim will be made many times in the story to many different recipients.

My first charge addresses HPCC's use of an embedded catheter without showing medical necessity. Shortly after arriving at HPCC, the doctor placed an indwelling urinary catheter without medical justification or to explain possible future medical ramifications that may result from their doing so to either my wife or me. The medical profession recognizes catheter-related problems due to indwelling urinary catheters (IUC).

One of the most common and severe complications with urinary catheters is a urinary tract infection (UTI), a 'catheter-associated urinary tract infection' or CAUTI, that can lead to urosepsis and septicemia. Disorders are common because a urethral catheter inoculates organisms into the bladder and promotes colonization by providing a surface for bacterial adhesion and causing mucosal irritation. A urinary catheter is the most critical risk factor for bacteriuria which usually occurs in patients with a catheter for 2 to 10 days.

A CAUTI is the most common nosocomial infection in hospitals and nursing homes, making up 80% of all institutionally gotten conditions. A CUTI is considered to be a complicated UTI and is the most common complication associated with long-term catheter use. CAUTIs may occur at least twice yearly in patients with long-term indwelling catheters requiring hospitalization.

They are associated with increased urosepsis, septicemia, and mortality. Urosepsis can result from a UTI, leading to generalized sepsis and death from severe UTIs. Mortality is more than three times higher in catheterized than in non-catheterized individuals. Confusion or unexplained fever may be the only symptoms of catheter-related CAUTI.

Beth exhibited extended periods of confusion, which the nursing home should have suspected might be coming from a CAUTI. In the above reference to septicemia, she was hospitalized on 8 November 2017 with a severe UTI. The CD identified the growth in the culture as septicemia, a condition that cannot be treated with regular prescription drugs. The standard treatment was to insert a PIC line in her arm and administer ten days of anti-bacterial medication. She was transferred to a rehab facility so their nurses could administer the daily injections.

Sepsis is a life-threatening illness caused by your body's response to an infection. Your immune system protects you from many diseases and disorders, but it is possible to go into overdrive in response to an infection. Sepsis develops when the immune system releases chemicals into the bloodstream to fight infection, causing inflammation. Sepsis is more common in seniors, especially those exposed to invasive devices, such as intravenous catheters—the most common condition that causes sepsis in seniors is urinary tract infections.

Staff convenience is a common reason for indwelling catheters, which many government organizations, including Medicare, condemn. There is the belief that it is more convenient for nursing homes to place a catheter rather than take the patient out of bed several times a day to change bedsheets and clothing, help her use a bedpan or walk to the bathroom, and change diapers. Nursing homes should never use these reasons to catheterize patients. Many medical facilities continue to do many unnecessary urinary catheterizations.

Despite the everyday use of catheters and the well-known risks of complications associated with urinary catheters, patients are not asked to sign a written consent that shows the advantages and disadvantages of urinary catheters. Rarely are patients informed verbally of the risks of urinary catheters.

It is a known fact that, in some cases, repeated UTIs will lead to kidney failure. Repeated UTIs often turn into pyelonephritis which is an inflammation of the kidney. Inflammation in the kidney worsens renal tissues seriously and thus causes kidney damage. Chronic kidney disease causes no apparent symptoms in the early stage. Without a prompt diagnosis, chronic kidney problems progress to an end state of kidney failure and eventually death.

The above describes why indwelling urinary catheters should not be used. Following is documentation that the nursing home acted recklessly, disregarding Medicare's mandated instruction on using indwelling urinary catheters. (Here, I quoted the mandates in CMS 20068, which I have previously detailed.)

In summary, HPCC needed a baseline care plan to present, in writing, to the resident or their representative. Despite the resident having no clinical condition requiring an indwelling urinary catheter, HPCC inserts one without discussion with the resident or their representative.

A contributing cause of Beth's death was continuing severe urinary tract infections (UTIs), which eventually shut down her kidney function. In the opinion of her urologist, the above-documented harmful effects of an indwelling urinary catheter embedded by HPCC in reckless disregard for Medicare procedure was a contributing factor to her numerous serious UTIs, which eventually shut down her kidneys, resulting in her death.

To quote CDC, "UTIs are the most common type of health-care-associated infections and are mostly caused by the placement or presence of a catheter in the urinary tract."

In the last two years of her life, she made twenty-seven trips to the hospital with suspected UTIs and was admitted twelve times with serious UTIs. The CDC further states, "Repeated UTIs will lead to kidney failure."

The second charge addressed the dehydration issue. On 18 June 2017, Beth was admitted to HPCC from the hospital for the skilled nursing needed while recovering from a fractured tibia. At admittance, her BUN level was 15. In July, a turgor test I performed showed Beth to be dehydrated, a diagnosis confirmed by the nursing staff. Getting her to drink more failed to improve her dehydration; she needed to be IV rehydrated, a procedure agreed to by the charge nurse.

The nurse could not initiate the process because Beth's veins kept collapsing, and HPCC did not have a nurse capable of inserting an IV line. As her BUN level increased, a sign of severe dehydration and possible UTI, I requested the PA send her to the ER to rehydrate, which she discouraged. Eventually, HPCC located a nurse who could insert an IV line to start rehydration, but it was too late.

Beth had been experiencing confusion and memory loss for weeks with fatigue and weakness symptoms. In the elderly, these are symptoms of dehydration and the possibility of a urinary tract infection.

Every UTI is a byproduct of dehydration and vice versa. With urinary infections in the elderly, a recurring problem in nursing homes, they must perform urine tests monthly to prevent them. On 28 July, during a visit to her ortho surgent, the nurses found Beth limp, and she kept falling asleep in her wheelchair. They recognized she was having a medical problem and for me to notify HPCC when she returned. HPCC had no response to my telling them of their concern.

On 29 July, I received a call from HPCC informing me Beth was found in a non-responsive state and was rushed to the hospital emergency room. Upon arrival, the ER doctors started aggressive rehydration through intravenous fluid insertion. She was also diagnosed with a UTI and pneumonia and remained hospitalized for four days. A stay was necessitated by HPCC's failure to adhere to standard operating procedures to prevent resident dehydration.

Dehydration results when too much water is lost from the body. The organs, cells, and tissues do not function as they should, leading to dangerous complications. If not corrected immediately, it could cause shock or a non-responsive state. Symptoms of severe dehydration are a medical emergency and should be treated by a medical professional immediately.

Seniors should be immediately treated even if they are experiencing symptoms of mild dehydration. Mild to moderate dehydration symptoms are sleepiness, fatigue, weakness, and disorientation, which Beth experienced before her hospital admission. Dehydration will also shut down vital organs. Beth was in a non-responsive state for at least three hours or more.

There is some concern about why the staff did not send Beth to the ER when they found her non-responsive rather than waiting for the doctor to tell them to do so. A non-responsive state is when a person does not respond to any stimuli. While in this state, the brain does not receive enough oxygen to sustain its normal metabolism.

Out of all the organs, a lack of oxygen is the most dangerous to the brain. Immediate medical attention is required to restore their oxygen supply, making the delay in transporting Beth to the ER even more critical. If a condition diminishes the amount of oxygen the brain receives, the situation might lead to brain hypoxia.

The prognosis of brain hypoxia depends on how long the brain is deprived of oxygen and whether the oxygen has been cut off entirely. If the brain has received too little oxygen for only a brief period, the symptoms might disappear once the brain gets enough oxygen again, and the patient can fully recover. More commonly, patients will experience memory problems.

Furthermore, we do not know how long Beth's oxygen may have been shut off while in a non-responsive state, but we do know that when Beth came around, from that time on, she experienced short-term memory loss. Dehydration is a significant cause of decreased mental acuity and associated memory loss, especially as you age. Dehydration can cause profound glucose levels and blood volume changes, especially when severe. These changes can be powerful enough to cause confusion, memory loss, and other dementia-like side effects.

Extreme or prolonged dehydration may cause severe cognitive impairment, delirium, permanent brain damage, or death, reports the *Mayo Clinic*. These are early warning signs of brain damage developing during the dehydration crisis if it is not treated immediately. I contend that the facility disregarded notification through Beth's representative and blood tests that she was dehydrated and did not have a nurse on staff capable of inserting an IV line for rehydration. It is also my contention that the delay in transporting Beth to the ER could have been a deciding factor as to how long her brain remained without oxygen and thus contributed to her resulting short-term memory loss.

My final charge, which I am not sure is applicable in these proceedings, has to do with what has been referred to as 'nursing home eviction.' On Saturday, 29 July 2017, Beth was rushed, by ambulance, to the hospital emergency room in a non-responsive state due to severe dehydration resulting from HPCC's negligence.

On 1 August, after a four-day hospital stay, she was denied re-entry to HPCC because there was no bed available, and I had not signed a 'bed hold' form not sent to the hospital, as per HPCC policy. After spending 60 days at HPCC and being rushed to the hospital due to their negligence, she was refused re-entry. A review of HPCC's census for that date shows that many Medicare beds were available, and she was not readmitted because she required too much care. I had one day to find another nursing home to accept Beth.

I want to quote an article entitled "Feds Seek to Stop Illegal Nursing Home Evictions." It states that discharges and evictions lead the yearly complaints that state ombudspersons receive. The report listed reasons a facility can legally evict a resident, and Beth did not meet any of them. The CMS states that once someone becomes a resident, '"it should be rare' for that facility to say later that it cannot meet that individual's needs.

The AARP said, "We appreciate that CMS plans to examine and mitigate the illegal discharge—or dump—of federally funded long-term care facilities residents." In another AARP article entitled, 'Nursing Homes: Stop Dumping Patients,' they give an example of a resident who had been in a nursing facility for an extended period and was sent to the hospital for an evaluation. When the hospital cleared her to return on the same day, the nursing home refused to take her back.

This was an example of what the AARP states: "The problem of patient dumping is one of the most troubling complaints of nursing home residents throughout the country." This is a form of abuse by nursing homes that dump these patients, especially Medicaid patients, to fill their beds with 'better' residents. The following quotation in the same article applies explicitly to Beth's situation.

"To maximize profit through decreased staffing, unscrupulous nursing facilities try to illegally evict the residents who are the neediest of staff time and require the greatest levels of care."

"One such method is hospital dumping. When a resident is temporarily hospitalized, the facility gives away the resident's bed and refuses to readmit the resident after they are medically cleared."

To quote from HPCC's 'Resident Handbook.' The resident or designee can hold the bed if the resident is transferred to the hospital by the following procedure.

"Upon patient transfer out of the facility, nursing will provide a copy of the Bed Hold Process in the transfer packet and contact the patient or patient representative to verbally notify them HPCC will contact them to discuss the Bed Hold."

HPCC never contacted me, or, as per the Case Manager, a Bed Hold Process form was not included in the transfer package. It is readily apparent that the nursing home did not want Beth back because of her extraordinary level of care and accomplished that aim by not including the Bed Hold Process form in her transfer package. The home was guilty of 'patient dumping.'

Chapter 16
Attorney Dissatisfaction

On 13 August, I e-mailed my attorney, telling him it had been three weeks since we talked, at which time he committed to keeping me updated on the case. I sent nine questions requesting case updates which he could answer by e-mail or in one of his suggested conference calls. As of 26 August, I was still awaiting a response to my e-mail.

I have reached my wit's end with my present attorney and started making inquiries with other law firms to see if they would be interested in taking over the litigation of my case. Despite my attorney's commitment to keeping me updated on the matter, he has failed to do so. I realize it is a complex task to change an attorney this late in the case, but if a new attorney is willing to accept all involved in such a more, I will make a move.

Still waiting to hear from my counsel, I talked to a local attorney about taking over the case. We talked for forty-five minutes, more than I spoke to my attorney in two years. He explained the ramifications associated with my case. He said it is exceedingly tricky for another attorney to take over an already-in-litigation issue. It comes down to the time it would take for a new attorney to get familiar with the case, and then having to share the damage award makes it not economically feasible to take the chance.

The reasoning being the fired attorney will have a lien or claim against the case to recover the fair and reasonable value of the time he spent on the subject; this lien may take the form of a percentage of the damage award. So why spend the time on the case to properly handle it if he must give up a hefty fee to the earlier lawyer?

He informed me that his biggest complaint about the legal profession is that an attorney does not respond to clients' repeated emails and phone calls or answer their questions. He said their non-response is annoying and prevents clients from working as a team to resolve the issue. I told him I felt like I was in the dark and was constantly begging for information about the status of the case.

He once again said what I already knew, "An attorney must return a client's calls promptly." He wished me luck dealing with my present counsel but said he was not interested in taking the case. He did inform me that I should not be hunting for an estate attorney but a probate attorney.

Following my attorney's instructions that I find an estate attorney, I spent weeks trying to find one, only to learn I was wasting my time and shorting the ninety-day time frame I had to file for being the new plaintiff in the lawsuit. He referred me to a probate attorney I contacted and had an appointment the following week.

He told me to continue with my present counsel and hope it works out. Although my attorney has violated many of the Rules Regulating Florida Bar rules dealing with Diligence and Communication, there is absolutely nothing I can do about it. Under Rule 4-1.4 Communications, it states that:

Keep the client informed about the status of the matter. Promptly comply with reasonable requests for information. Reasonably consult with the client about how the client's objectives are accomplished. Communication between the lawyer and the client is necessary for the client to participate in the representation effectively.

The lawyer's regular contact with clients will minimize the occasions when a client needs to request information concerning the representation. When a client makes a reasonable request for information, it requires prompt compliance with the request. If a quick response is not possible, the lawyer, or a member of the lawyer's staff, acknowledges receipt of the request and advises the client when they may expect a reply.

It is okay for the Florida Bar to set up these rules, but there is no way the client can get recourse if the attorney chooses to ignore them. If the client calls the attorney out on disregarding the rules, their response can be, "If you aren't happy with my representation, then find a new attorney," knowing this is an almost impossible task.

Chapter 17
Probate

On 29 August, I met with a probate attorney, a hire I must make to keep the lawsuit active. An estate means everything of monetary value; in Beth's case, since she has no assets in her name, it will be the damage award from the lawsuit. Since she is no longer alive, her estate collects all the money, and I now become her representative, and the medical negligence case becomes a wrongful death case upon her passing.

To become a wrongful death case, one must prove fault. A description is that the decedent did not die immediately from the negligent act of the nursing home but consciously suffered from severe pain before passing away. One must prove the following elements of a wrongful death case:

Duty of Care: The defendant owed a duty of care to the deceased person and breached that duty of care owed to the plaintiff.

Causation: The plaintiff must show that the defendant's action directly caused the wrongful death. Remember this, for it becomes a principal factor in pursuing a wrongful death case. HPCC had a 'duty of care' to protect the plaintiff against injuries while in their care. By wantonly ignoring Medicare mandates about the insertion of an indwelling catheter, and the probable cause of such catheter subjecting the plaintiff to severe and painful urinary tract infections, HPCC did not meet the duty of care element.

I contend that the medical records prove the elements of negligence supported by a 'preponderance of evidence' that her wrongful death resulted from negligent and willful omission on the defendant's part.

On the internet, I researched "What Are the Main Duties of a Probate Attorney." Every will must go through the probate process. In our case, I do not have the original will, only a copy. There is no other option than to treat

Beth as having died 'intestate,' meaning she died without having a will. All the community property passes to the spouse with or without a will.

The primary duties of the probate attorney are he initially files the probate petition to appoint someone as the personal representative, which would be me. He must then publish a notice of filing a partition for letters in a newspaper of general circulation.

Creditors then have 120 days from issuing letters to file a creditor's claim in the probate to receive payment. In Beth's case, there are no creditors, but the time frame stands. The probate process takes six months because the personal representative must go through 120 days to let creditors file claims. At the end of that period, file a notice and petition for final distribution.

To get to the 120 days, the client's attorney must sign and file the partition with the court. The court then assigns a hearing date, and depending on how busy the court's calendar is, it typically takes about 40 days. If everything is in order at the hearing, the court grants the partition, admits the will to probate, and issues letters testamentary to the personal representative.

At this point, the 120 days for a creditor to file claims begins. I can do nothing to reduce the 120 days because it is a statutory requirement. An attorney is essential because the probate procedures are so complex. Because of the complexity, a process that you expect to take two to three months may run between 8 and 12 months.

If the original medical malpractice case had concluded before her death, none of the above probate procedures would have been necessary. The settled funds would have gone directly to her without probate. Her death does not reduce the damage cap but increases the litigation cost by thousands.

On 29 July, I met with my probate attorney, who educated me on the probate process. He must prepare the documents to present to the court naming me as the personal representative of Beth. Document prep will take about a week, but court approval may take four months. Once I am named, a notice must be placed in the newspaper that anyone with a debt claim against Elizabeth must submit it to the probate attorney. Calling me the personal representative and the lawsuit can run concurrently.

My attorney did not tell me that a probate attorney must be retained as soon as possible after the plaintiff's death because the case cannot resume until the court appoints me. If you recall, my attorney previously e-mailed me telling me to hire an estate attorney. I learned from other sources that I should have been searching for a probate attorney, not an estate attorney.

A significant difference between the two. He should have informed me that I needed to retain one expeditiously. I had ninety days after the plaintiff's death to send documents concerning probate to the court, or the case would have gone into abeyance and have to be reinstituted.

In off-the-record discussions, the probate attorney almost recommended I seek new counsel. He agreed that it is unheard of that I do not have a copy of my contract and the contingency fee agreement. My present attorney, by law, is bound to submit signed copies to me, and requests for documents have yet to be responsive. I now await my next appointment with the probate attorney when I get an estimate of his fee.

The case now goes into a holding pattern until the court appoints me as Beth's representative, and it could take up to a month to get court approval. What pisses me off is that this process could have started the week after Beth's death if my attorney had taken the time to inform me of the importance of getting a probate attorney. His incompetence becomes increasingly evident as I get to talk to other attorneys.

On 5 September, I signed eleven forms necessary to submit to the court, making me Beth's representative. The attorney must submit these forms within ninety days of her death, and the probate attorney will keep on this process to ensure the court signs off on the documents before 5 October, the day of her death, ninety days ago.

This stage of the lawsuit is interesting. By dying, wrongful death will become a count in the amended complaint. In addition, it is now necessary for a probate attorney to be hired to file a Petition for Administration. In paragraph one, the petitioner has an interest in the above estate as the decedent's surviving spouse and nominated Personal Representative under the last will, filed with the probate court.

Paragraph five states that John is qualified under the laws of the State of Florida to serve as a personal representative of the decedent's estate and is entitled to preference in appointment as a personal representative because the individual was named as Personal Representative under the decedent's last will. This form and four others will be filed with the court, and the lawsuit can continue after the court has approved me as a personal representative.

By Beth dying, I now incur a minimum charge of $3,000 plus costs for ordinary services for the probate attorney to file the court documents. I also agreed to pay for extraordinary services on six-minute segments at rates from $50 to $400 per hour. I know the minimum probate service costs but not the maximum.

On 29 August, I got answers to the questions I submitted to my attorney on 13 August. He informed me that an amendment to the complaint is better than responding to the defendant's Motion to Dismiss. He will revise the original complaint to address the items detailed in the defense's MTD.

The plaintiff may amend their complaint only by the defendant's consent, but the court will allow the plaintiff to amend the complaint unless it prejudices the defendant. My attorney can take no action until I am appointed personal representative and become the new plaintiff.

Chapter 18
Ring Theft

Having downtime waiting for the judge to grant my request to be appointed Personal Representative, I sent Beth's $4700 wedding ring to New York to appraise it for sale. A few days later, I got a message from the appraiser saying they were not interested in the ring and were returning it. I could not understand why they had no interest in a .76-weight diamond. When they returned the ring, I inspected it and found it did not match the diamond appraisal description on my purchase document.

The discrepancy noticed immediately was that the ring returned was a four-prong mount, and the ring bought was a six-prong mount. I immediately called the appraiser to see if they had returned the right ring. They informed me it was the right ring, and the diamond was a fake. I was stunned. How could it be fake? After careful review, I determined that the ring was stolen while she was in nursing care.

Beth entered the assisted living facility in May 2018 wearing a $4700 diamond wedding ring. When she died in a hospice in July of 2019, based on the ring returned to me, she was wearing a $20 fake. It is suspected that her ring was taken and replaced with an almost identical imitation sometime during her last rehab stay. While in this facility, where she spent 48 days in the memory care unit while getting physical therapy, the attendants had time to study the ring and obtain a fake remarkably like the actual ring.

While in this rehab, her rings had to be removed and put back on. In her condition, and since the rings looked the same, she could not determine whether she got back her real ring or a fake. Whoever took the ring could match the fake ring to the actual ring, so I suspect this may not have been their first such theft. Much thought went into this theft. If they had taken the ring outright, it would have resulted in a theft investigation by the facility.

However, by replacing the ring with a fake diamond, there would be no reason to believe an 82-year-old sick, and the confused resident would notice any difference between the real and fake ring. Under these circumstances, the theft would only be seen once the resident died, which could be years, and the heir tried to sell what they believed to be the diamond ring.

I blame myself for not taking the ring when she was in these facilities, but it is difficult to ask your wife, who has worn the ring for sixty years, to surrender her wedding ring because someone giving her health care may steal it.

I have no evidence to substantiate my conclusions, but circumstantial evidence proves my findings correct. It is challenging to imagine an aide employed to give health care would take advantage of a sick, confused, and dying patient, but thieves do not consider the condition of their victims.

The theft still bothers me, and I still think about how they could have gotten away with it by just taking the ring and not trying to replace it with a fake. My wife or I would have never noticed the ring was missing. When she died, and there was no wedding ring, I would have assumed she had lost the ring and accepted that reasoning. Thinking it might have been stolen would not have entered the picture.

On 9 October, I phoned in a theft complaint to the County Sheriff. A deputy came to the house, reviewed the case, and said there was nothing they could do about it. He reasoned that not knowing how long ago the theft occurred would prevent them from trying to find the ring. His second reason for not being a case is my wife's condition.

With her being in memory care, there is always the possibility that she agreed to trade her real ring for the fake. He did give the complaint a case number, but there is no case, and I will have to live with the $4700 loss.

After stewing for a few months thinking about the ring theft, I wrote to the rehab center, where I suspected the ring was stolen.

Elizabeth was moved from the hospital to MCHC on 24 April wearing a $4700 diamond wedding ring and died on 8 July 2019 wearing a $20 fake diamond ring. Her ring was stolen during that period, but the theft was not discovered until hospice returned her ring to me.

Reviewing her care from the time she entered MCHC wearing a diamond wedding ring and her stay in the hospital before going to hospice, the only place in that scenario where someone would have removed her ring would have been at MCHC. While there, I know aides removed her rings many times to bathe her or for other purposes, but they removed them. For someone to have time to study the actual ring and find a fake match, it would have to be in a facility where she would be a resident for an extended period. Neither the hospital nor hospice meets those criteria.

The theft of the ring took much thought to accomplish. Getting the ring off her finger, replacing it with a look-alike fake, knowing an 82-year-old resident in memory care would never be able to recognize the difference, and going on the basis the resident may live a long time before the theft would be discovered. Elizabeth was in MCHC for forty-eight days, during which the above scenario could have happened.

During that stay, her $4700 diamond wedding ring was removed by a caregiver and replaced with a fake replica. I thus seek $2318, the present-day value placed on the ring by a diamond appraiser. As expected, I am still waiting for an answer. So, this ends the stolen ring saga.

Chapter 19
Case Resumption

On 7 October, the 'Order Admitting Will to Probate and Appointing Personal Representative' was received by the probate attorney and sent to me. The signature date met the ninety-day time frame. I informed my attorney that the court had appointed me Elizabeth's representative, and he could now prepare and send his suggested amendment to the complaint. Once again, I requested a copy of the signed contract and contingency agreement.

On 5 November, for only the third time in two and a half years, I got to speak on the phone with my attorney. He informed me that the amended complaint was being prepared and would incorporate more specific allegations to rebut June MTD and send it to the court soon. I asked that I be told when it was filed and that I would be copied.

With HPCC being a Medicare facility, I asked him if we could sue in federal court rather than civil court, thus bypassing the Sovereign Immunity Statutes regarding damages. The answer is no, the reasoning being. No provision of section 768.28 of the Sovereign Immunity Statutes or any other area of the Florida Statutes shall be construed to waive the state's immunity or any of its agencies from suit in federal court.

The Eleventh Amendment guarantees such immunity. The first part of the amendment reads: "The judicial power of the United States shall not be construed to extend to any suit in law or equity," which is the section of the amendment which grants sovereign immunity entities from being sued in federal court.

He confirmed that a wrongful death case does not have different damage caps. Florida Statutes state that neither the state nor its agencies shall be liable to pay a claim or a judgment by anyone who exceeds $200,000 for pain and suffering. In Florida, if you suffer a catastrophic personal injury, including death, due to a negligent act of a state agency, which includes the nursing home in question, and even if your medical expenses to treat the careless act exceed $200,000, the most one can recover is a maximum $200,000 as per the statute caps on damages.

The statutes define pain. There is physical pain and suffering, the pain of the plaintiff's actual physical pain and discomfort that the claimant had endured before their death. There is mental pain and suffering, any negative emotion a victim suffers because of having to take the physical pain and trauma resulting from the health care negligence.

As described, Beth endured physical and mental pain, thus establishing a $200,000 judgment claim. The loss of consortium damages typically relates to the injuries' impact on the plaintiff's relationship with their spouse—loss of companionship. The description of how Beth spent the last year of her life in assisted living, memory care, the hospital, a nursing home, and hospice meets all the requirements for the loss of consortium. Still, that loss is included in the $200,000 maximum damage award per statute.

After receiving the amended complaint, my attorney thought the defendant would want to abate the action and move to arbitration. The defendant's logical next step would be to make a settlement offer rather than be stuck with the arbitration costs.

Come 16 November, I had not heard from my attorney about whether he had filed the amendment. However, I decided to take another approach to keep informed on the case's progress. On 15 October, I submitted a notarized 'Registration Agreement to View Records,'' allowing me to access all the legal documents submitted to the court. Case review showed the attorneys had introduced 25 papers, many of which I was unaware had been offered.

I wondered why my attorney had not directed me to this site immediately after the case was assigned a court case number. On 15 November, court records revealed that my attorney had filed the amended complaint with the court on 8 November. He did not tell me it had been filed nor sent me a copy as per his commitment.

On 4 October, my attorney submitted a letter to the court naming me Beth's representative, and on 8 October, the court granted the substitution of parties. In a teleconference with the court and the opposing counsel on 1 October, my attorney notified the court that the plaintiff was deceased. He will file an amended complaint naming a substitute personal representative.

None of the actions mentioned in this paragraph were ever conveyed to me by my counsel. I also discovered that the court had scheduled a 9 December hearing to discuss why my attorney had not addressed the MTD filed by the defendant. The hearing may have been the incentive my attorney needed to submit the amended complaint, which served to cancel the scheduled hearing.

In reviewing the 'Motion for Leave of Court to File Amended Complaint,' The amendment, excluding the cover letter, was 24 pages long and named the two defendants, the nursing home and the home's administrator. The first paragraph, entitled 'Amended Complaint and Demand for Jury Trial,' states the plaintiff, John, as personal representative of the estate of Elizabeth, deceased, by and through undersigned counsel, and now files the Amended Complaint against Defendants listing the following allegations.

The following 22 pages of the amendment look like a standard format with the names and dates inserted to fit the case, and it took LGF 120 days to insert the pertinent data into the traditional form. His reason for the delay in answering the MTD was that he incorporated information that would make the defendant want to abate the claim and go to arbitration after receiving the amended complaint.

From what I can read, the submission was just a standard document, and the only amendment to the original complaint appeared to be a notification of the plaintiff's death. For instance, one section states, "During Elizabeth's residency at HPCC, the employees and agents under the direct control of the defendants were negligent in the following ways." It then lists 23 "Failing-to-dos" covering two and a half pages of the complaint.

These were the same issues described in the original complaint. Then under the heading General Allegations Applicable to Defendants, there are six pages detailing the same allegations described in the General Allegations section, only in a different language.

The document then outlines Count I DEPRIVATION OR INFRINGEMENT OF RESIDENT'S RIGHTS.

The first article states, "The plaintiff incorporates and re-alleges paragraphs one through 28 above as though fully set forth here." It again describes what has already been portrayed twice in the proceeding complaint. Count II NEGLIGENCE.

It states once again, "The Plaintiff incorporates and re-alleges paragraphs one (1) through twenty-eight (28) above as though fully set forth" and then goes on again to describe all the charges previously stated. Count III NEGLIGENCE duplicates Count II and likewise explains the complaints already detailed. In conclusion, after 23 pages of repeated allegations, the final reason for the amended complaint is stated.

WHEREFORE, Plaintiff JOHN, as personal representative of the estate of Elizabeth, demands all damages which he is entitled to recover under the Florida Wrongful Death Act, including loss of companionship, care, comfort, society, and mental pain and suffering from the date of injury to Elizabeth and into the future, with costs against Defendant and a trial by jury.

The contingency fee for this lawsuit is for the attorney's knowledge of what forms to compile and submit to the court. Looking at the amendment, he did not have to be creative in detailing the allegations since the revision used were the same as I described two years ago in my interrogatories.

It took 24 pages to tell the defendant they screwed up, and we expect them to pay for their negligence. As promised, my attorney still needs to furnish me with that information or a copy to inform me when he filed the amended complaint. I am not letting him know I now have access to all filed court documents and have already obtained a copy of the amended complaint.

On 12 November 2019, I finally received a copy of the contract signed with LGF in August 2017, stating they had furnished me a copy at signing. The contract is MEDICAL MALPRACTICE/NURSING HOME NEGLIGENCE AUTHORITY TO REPRESENT (Contingent Attorney Fee Agreement).

Under the section Attorney Fees, their fee is 40% of the gross recovery through trial before a judge or arbitrated before an arbitration panel.

The following paragraph states, "It is further expressly understood and agreed that this employment is upon a contingent fee basis. If no recovery is made by suit, settlement, or otherwise, the client will not be indebted to attorneys for any sum whatsoever for attorneys' fees."

"Provided, however, should the client discharge the attorneys retained herein, then said attorney will have the right to claim payment from any suit settlement, whether made through client effort or any subsequently included attorneys. Still, they may be entitled to amounts based on the value of their services provided during their representation (quantum merit) and not on the percentages in this agreement."

"In other words, if I should fire my present attorney and hire a new one, the fired attorney would still be entitled to payment from the settlement equal to the value of their services while representing me. This hang-up makes it challenging to retain a new attorney since he would be in a difficult position to determine what contingency fee would be paid to the fired attorney."

Under the section, Costs states, "Client agrees to pay from the net proceeds of any recovery the costs of investigation or other reasonable expenses to prepare and prosecute this action." Under the Clients' Rights, the client is entitled to get an expense summary to date when requested, a request my attorney is reluctant to provide, saying LGF will give it at the end of the lawsuit. Based on the Clients' Rights, it is illegal to prevent the client from seeing what expenses have been billed to the case.

Under the section General Provisions, there is an interesting statement, "The undersigned Client at this moment acknowledges that my undersign attorneys may petition the Court for approval of these fees, which exceed the limitation of Rule 4.4-1.5, and I hereby consent to their representation to the Court that I have been unable to obtain an attorney of my choice because of the limitations outlined in subdivision 4F of the above-referenced rule."

The rule states that the max contingency fee for a sovereign immunity lawsuit is 25%. However, by my inability to find an attorney wanting to take the case for that percentage, I have agreed to pay the 40%.

Also, under this section, "The undersigned Client, before signing this agreement, received and read the Statement of Client's Rights, and understands each of the rights set forth therein. The undersigned client signed the Statement of Client's Rights and received a signed copy to keep and refer to while represented by the undersigned attorney."

I did not sign nor have a copy.

Two days later, I got the 'Clients Rights Statement' without explaining why it was not provided after being signed by LGF two years ago.

Chapter 20
Review of Court Cases

I researched sovereign immunity court cases and found an exciting issue concerning Florida's statute limiting damage caps for non-economic damages.

In a hospital lawsuit, the jury awarded the plaintiff $4,700,000 in damages, of which $2,000,000 was for past pain and suffering. The court, however, limited the non-economic damage award to the caps provided in Section 766.118, $200,000, and reduced the 4-million-dollar verdict citing the 'limitations on non-economic damages for negligence.'

The plaintiff challenged, and the court rejected her contention that section 766.118 caps on non-economic damages in medical negligence actions were unconstitutional. The plaintiff appealed to the district court.

The district court held that statutory caps on non-economic damage awards in personal injury medical malpractice actions are unconstitutional. Relying on a 2014 Florida case, the cap on wrongful death non-economic damages in section 766.118 violated the Equal Protection Clause of Florida's Constitution. They directed the trial court to reinstate the total damage award as found by the jury. The defendant appealed to the Supreme Court.

In June 2017, the Supreme Court decided these caps 'arbitrarily reduce damage awards for plaintiffs who suffer the most drastic injuries.' It struck any statutory limits on non-economic damages in medical malpractice lawsuits. The court affirmed the district court's decision.

It held that caps on personal injury and non-economic damages in medical negligence actions provided in section 766.118 violate the Equal Protection Clause of the Florida Constitution. I will summarize the court decision because the reasoning used by the court could also apply to sovereign immunity cases.

The court stated that section 766.118 has the effect of saving a modest amount for many by imposing devasting costs on a few—those who are most grievously injured, those who sustain the most significant damage, and loss for whom non-economic damages are based upon the existence of the cap on damages. Under the Equal Protection Clause of the Florida Constitution, we held that to reduce damages in this fashion is not only arbitrary but irrational, and we conclude that it "offends the fundamental notion of equal justice under the law."

They also concluded that the cap; on non-economic damages "Bears no rational relationship to a legitimate state objective, they failing the rational basis test." The Florida legislature's purpose in enacting the statute was to address the medical malpractice insurance crisis. The legislature asserted that the increase in medical malpractice insurance premiums was detrimental to physicians and caused them to leave, retire or refuse to perform substantial risk procedures, thereby limiting the availability of health care.

However, the court determined that available data did not support the legislature's findings on the existence of a medical malpractice crisis. The opinion declared that even if the legislature's results were accurate, section 766.118 still violates Florida's Equal Protection Clause because the available evidence does not show a rational relationship between a cap on non-economic damages and alleviation of the crises. There is a lack of evidence showing a direct correlation between caps on reduced malpractice premiums.

The Florida court added the Texas Supreme Court's statement, "In the context of persons catastrophically injured by medical negligence, we believed it is unreasonable and arbitrary to limit their recovery in a speculative experiment to determine whether liability insurance rates will decrease."

Furthermore, the Florida court opinion asserts that even if a medical malpractice crisis existed when the statute was enacted, "Conditions can change which remove or negate the justification for a law, transforming what may have once been reasonable into arbitrary and irrational legislation."

The court then stated, after reviewing current data, "No rational basis exists to justify the continued application of non-economic damage caps of section 766.118." Caps on non-economic damages serve no purpose but to punish the most grievously injured arbitrarily."

The court also saw that "The only asserted legitimate State interest is the alleviation of rising medical malpractice insurance premiums paid by affected doctors." However, "There is no mechanism to assure the savings are passed on from the insurance companies to the doctors." Thus, the court concluded there was no evidence of a continuing medical malpractice crisis that would justify the arbitrary application of the statutory cap in a wrongful death case.

The court's final opinion was that the district court's view that 766.118 was unconstitutional was upheld.

The Supreme Court said, "We agree with the district court and hold that the caps in 766.118 violate equal protection under the rational basis test. The caps apply to the plaintiff because the arbitrary reduction of compensation without regard to the severity of the injury does not bear a rational relationship to the legislature' stated interest in addressing the medical malpractice crisis."

Therefore, we held that caps on personal injury non-economic damages provided n section 766.118 violate the Equal Protection Clause of the Florida Constitution. However, a dissenting opinion stated.

Most of the court disregards and ignores all the legislature's work and fact-finding. Under our constitutional system, the legislature and not this court is entitled to make laws as a matter of policy based upon the facts it finds. The legislature's task is to decide whether a medical malpractice crisis exists, whether a medical malpractice crisis has abated, and whether the Florida Statutes should be amended accordingly. For most of this court to decide that a problem no longer exists, if it ever existed, so it can change a statute and policy it dislikes, improperly interjects the judiciary into a legislative function.

This Statue and the Sovereign Immunity Statute setting damage caps for malpractice evolved in the late 80s and 90s. The legislature felt that protecting medical providers from escalating malpractice lawsuits and liability insurance rates would bring more physicians to practice in the state and lower healthcare costs by reducing malpractice insurance premiums.

Opponents, however, claim that neither of those benefits has happened, and the state has done more harm than good. Rather than bringing in good doctors, the statute has attracted physicians who have experienced malpractice suits elsewhere and has pointed to the fact that malpractice insurance and healthcare costs have continued to climb.

Despite the Supreme Court ruling that 766.118 was unconstitutional, the statute is still in the 2019 Florida Statutes. Thus, attorneys consider the following before deciding to take on a case.

Lawyers treat entities covered under the Sovereign Immunity statute like physicians not having medical malpractice insurance, a practice referred to as 'going bare.' A *USA TODAY* study found that 8.3% of Florida's licensed doctors go bare. Many physicians are licensed to practice in Florida after facing disciplinary action in other states.

Like sovereign immunity caps, doctors who do not carry medical malpractice insurance have no federal or Florida state laws requiring them to do so. The state allows said doctors to promise to pay $250,000 if the plaintiff wins the lawsuit. However, federal bankruptcy law creates a loophole. In contrast, the physician can file for bankruptcy instead of paying the damages, and the state medical board cannot discipline them.

By the 1980s, malpractice insurance premiums were so high that some doctors were retiring early or practicing elsewhere. The Tort Reform and Insurance Act of 1986 was supposed to solve this problem by changing insurance regulations. Inserted into the Act was Chapter 458, which allowed physicians to forgo medical malpractice insurance for the first time.

The law required the doctors to agree to satisfy any adverse medical malpractice judgment against them for up to $250,000. However, lawmakers created another by trying to fix one problem, whereas the most problematic doctors in the state had the most incentive to stop carrying medical malpractice insurance. One of the first things an attorney asks a potential client is whether the doctor has medical malpractice insurance; if not usually walks away.

Regarding increasing insurance rates, the most prominent physician-owned medical malpractice insurer in Florida states that one lawsuit will not necessarily increase insurance premiums, but a track record of problems can.

"Rates are increased in repose to a pattern of claim activity that identifies an individual practitioner as having a high-risk profile than the average physician."

The Florida legislators felt that protecting medical providers from escalating malpractice suits and liability insurance rates would encourage more physicians to practice in Florida and lower the cost of malpractice premiums. Opponents argue that neither of the benefits has accrued, and malpractice insurance and health care costs continue to rise despite the exemption steadily.

The constitutionality of the law has been challenged. Still, in 2000, the Florida Supreme Court upheld the exclusion as constitutional, saying, "the statute's disparate treatment of medical malpractice wrongful deaths does bear a rational relationship to the legitimate state interest of ensuring the accessibility of medical care to Florida residents by curtailing the skyrocketing medical malpractice insurance in Florida."

Chapter 21
Nursing Home Standards

HPCC was guilty of medical procedure malpractice, but I wondered how such misconduct would be discovered before a resident's death. Nursing homes are subject to inspections, but how can medical procedure malpractice be found if it does not occur while the inspector is in the facility or after the review has been completed? Inspections are to be conducted every 15 months, and many non-medical procedures can occur between inspections.

I was the one who discovered the malfeasance through medical research, but how many patients or their representatives know or have the time to do such research? How many nursing home malpractice suits are not filed because the aggrieved party needs to have the knowledge to review their medical care thoroughly?

Following is a review of the nursing home inspection process and the criteria for grading the home following the inspection.

A study conducted by the *USA Today* Network found that since 2013, state inspections have found 291 violations for failure to guarantee adequate and proper care. This broad category can include the most severe violation involving death. Beth received inadequate care, and even though she did not experience the result at HPCC, it was the contributing cause of her later death.

The study also found 215 incidents of nursing homes not following doctor's orders or blood work results. This finding corresponds with Beth's treatment, where the staff did not respond to blood tests or the patient's representative notification that the patient was severely dehydrated.

The Florida Agency for Health Care Administration (AHCA) routinely fines nursing homes, with the average fine from June 2012 through 2017 averaging $4500. Florida law sets the largest AHCA fine for a severe violation at $15,000. Compare this to the millions of dollars homes receive from taxpayer-funded Medicare programs each year.

The AHCA states that "Fines are generally enough to prompt facility improvement," saying, "It is not the amount of the fine; it's a fact of the fine that gets the facility to improve." However, a state senator disagreed, saying he is concerned that low fines hinder improvement.

He states, "Here is a reality of capitalism."

"If there is no financial disincentive, safety, and responsibility tend to become just bottom-line numbers." In other words, fines just become an accepted expense of doing business.

FAHA, which licenses and regulates nursing homes, rarely uses the most onerous sanctions. HPCC has had, during the period 2013 through 2017, one federal fine of $5,850. They had 33 violations cited in that period but no state fines.

To quote a FAHA official, "We are required by Florida law to take the least invasive, least intrusive licensure action that we can take under the circumstance. Our action will be reviewed and vetted in every situation, whether a small fine, a moratorium, or a suspension."

Federal Government fines are higher, with the average penalty in Florida in the above period being $27,000. By law, AHCA is to receive a copy of nursing home lawsuits, but only some lawyers comply, thus preventing prospective residents from reviewing a nursing home's lawsuit history.

How could the violation of medical procedures described in the complaint go unnoticed? The following regulations apply to nursing home inspections: NURSING HOME FEDERAL DEFICIENCY SEVERITY AND SCOPE.

Nursing homes certified to accept Medicare or Medicaid must meet specific federal requirements. The Agency for Health Care Administration conducts inspections for federal decertification. When a national deficiency is cited during a review, the fault is assigned a 'scope and severity' based on the finding.

Scope describes how many persons are affected by the deficiency: Isolated involves one or a limited number of residents or issues. Pattern involves more than a limited number of residents or problems and is usually a group, a unit, or a wing. Widespread involves many residents and may be pervasive or systematic.

Severity shows the level of harm to health or safety. Immediate Jeopardy is harmful or; potential damage occurring now. An actual injury has occurred. There is no real harm, but there is a potential for more than minimal harm; no actual harm occurred, and the potential for harm is minimal.

A grading system is used by the state and CMS to rate the seriousness of deficiencies found during an inspection. A 'deficiency' is a regulatory requirement the facility does not meet.

A nursing home graded as a level 1 on the severity chart shows that the facility's deficient practice has caused or is likely to cause severe injury, harm, impairment, or death and requires immediate action/correction. In our case, the pattern of the facility's practice shows a reasonable degree of predictability of similar actions, situations, procedures, or incidents occurring in the future if they do not fix them immediately. Level 1 is called Immediate Jeopardy.

For each deficiency, the survey team first decides the scope of the problem within the nursing home. It assigns an alphabetical severity and scope value using the letters A through L and determines whether the deficiency is isolated, pattern, or widespread. J shows it to be isolated Immediate Jeopardy and is the most severe deficiency, even though it applies to the fewest number of residents.

K is immediate pattern jeopardy but only affects a limited number of residents, and L is widespread. To determine a finding of Immediate Jeopardy, the inspector must look for the following components:

The first category is harm, having two options, actual or potential. The second part is Immediacy. The investigator looks to see if the harm or potential harm will occur soon if immediate action is not taken. The third part is Culpability, and the team will ask: Did the facility know about the situation, and if so, when did they know? Should the facility have known about the problem? Did the facility thoroughly investigate the circumstances? Did the facility implement corrective measures? Has the facility reevaluated the steps to ensure situation correction?

The team considers the facility's response to any harm or potential harm that meets the definition of Immediate Jeopardy. Just because the facility's staff says they did not know about a particular issue or situation does not excuse the facility from learning about and preventing Immediate Jeopardy.

The survey team uses their experience and knowledge to determine if the circumstances could have been predicted and should have been investigated to evaluate any prior indications or warnings about the jeopardy situation. Crises in which a facility did not have any previous indications or warnings are rare.

Let us take the events associated with the present lawsuit. If occurring during an inspection, would the inspector know about it unless informed by a resident or their representative? Only by the inspector seeing a resident with an embedded catheter could they inquire why it was being used and determine its Immediate Jeopardy resulting from continued use.

Let us start with the deficiency's scope, which would fall under the 'isolated involves only one resident.' How would the inspector know whether the practice was isolated to one resident, patterned involving a limited number of residents, or widespread and systematic?

Whether the discrepancy meets the components of Immediate Jeopardy is the finding as to whether it meets all three. It meets the potential Harm category by "The facility's failure to comply with requirements likely to cause severe injury, harm, impairment or death to an individual." An embedded catheter meets the criteria since catheters are known to cause UTIs, and frequent UTIs can cause kidney failure and death.

Criteria two is immediacy, whereby harm or potential harm will likely occur soon if immediate action is not taken. In our case, per Medicare mandates, the facility's failure to remove the catheter as soon as possible ensured the patient suffered continued UTIs. As for category three, Culpability, questions. Did the facility know about the situation, and when did they know it?

The answer is that the facility knew of the Medicare mandate against using a catheter as soon as they embedded it. As for the question, should the facility know about the situation? If they had read and followed Medicare mandates, they would have known that embedding a catheter violated Medicare directives. Based on the above, the facility would have gotten a grade of 1 J and have faced a stiff fine.

How would an inspection team know medical malpractice is occurring between inspections? How many residents or representatives would know an embedded catheter was against the Medicare mandate and that its continued use could result in kidney failure and death?

One must rely on the facility to give a resident proper contracted for competent medical care, which HPCC should have provided. The only recourse is to file a formal complaint with Medicare, making them aware of

HPCC's violation of Medicare mandates on catheter use. I plan to pursue how to file such a complaint.

Staffing is another nursing home problem. Beth's catheter embedding was not a medical necessity but was embedded to reduce the aide's workload of taking her to the bathroom or changing her diaper. Was this because the facility lacked aides and ran with available aide staffing? The only alternative was to reduce the aides' general workload—three factors affecting staff to residents.

Regulation: For Assisted Living facilities (ALF), Florida does not require a minimum staff based on the number of residents in the ALF. They only mandate adequate staffing to supervise residents and fulfill their service plan. However, nursing homes have more rigorous standards, which dictate RN and LPN staffing requirements, but there are no requirements for specific numbers of care aides.

Living Up to Standards: Most ALFs only live up to federal standards, but most states impose more significant standards. Studies show that understaffing is widespread in nursing and ALF facilities, and ratios are rarely met.

Cost: Money is another factor whereby residents with the most money can access facilities with better resident-to-staff ratios since high cost usually means enough employees to help residents properly. Studies have shown that nursing homes are notoriously understaffed, and more staff equals better care.

Insufficient staff numbers also mean high employee turnover and constant stress for employees. A resident has a substantial risk of having someone whose training could be better, or the resident may be cared for by someone exhausted and overworked.

I experienced the constant change of aides treating my wife in the nursing homes, so neither the aide nor the resident gets to know each other. The area has 24 ALF and 15 care facilities, with at least one hundred residents or patients. Staffing of RNs, LPNs, and aides at these facilities will become more complex and challenging as more facilities open.

In a Virginia study, one of the findings was that state surveyors could not determine if a nursing home or ALF meets federal staffing standards due to the vague definition of the term in the criteria, such as 'sufficient staff' and the subjective nature of the survey process. The same goes for Florida, which requires a facility to have adequate staffing to provide necessary health care to the residents and patients.

On 20 February 2020, the local newspaper featured a front-page article entitled 'Nursing homes could get less oversight.' The paper referred to the Florida Agency for Health Care Administration (ACHA) and mentioned that the agency cited three nursing homes with Class 1 violations, the most severe violation the agency can levy over the last three years. Current law would require the agency to inspect these homes every six months for two years. However, two bills considered in the Florida legislature would reduce inspections at problem nursing homes.

Part of the legislation would require the agency to do only one added review after a nursing home had been cited with a Class 1 or multiple Class 2 violations and cut AHCA inspection fines from $6000 to $3000. The AHCA is pushing legislation to allow the agency to spend less time in good healthcare facilities and more time inspecting problem facilities. The AHCA states that their resources are increasingly strained as the state's population and healthcare facilities increase.

The agency says, "We want to make sure that we can focus on higher risk and poor performing providers as we look at our workload."

A 2018 investigation by two local newspapers found that dozens of Florida's worst nursing homes have long records of not meeting state and federal standards and run with an insignificant risk that regulators will shut them down. At this writing, Florida had 695 nursing homes, 59 subject to the more intense two-year inspection cycle, with 52 having a below-average rating from the federal Centers for Medicare and Medicaid Services of 1.9 stars on a five-point scale.

These are the facilities the AHCA wants to concentrate its efforts on. The bill would allow the agency to extend inspection deadlines at highly rated facilities and emphasize poorly rated ones. Regardless of the proposed legislation, the AHCA would still have to follow federal requirements that mandate all nursing facilities be inspected every 15 months.

The requirement that AHCA ramp up oversight for nursing homes with serious violations became law in 2001, part of a divisive nursing home reform effort that also mandated increased staffing to give the long-term care industry increased protections against lawsuits. However, staffing has remained flat over the last six years, with the year 2015 staffing being 596 full-time employees and in 2019 rising to 597.

In that period, its healthcare providers' inspections have increased from 18,107 to 19,601, an 8% increase. Nursing home incidents increased by 7%, adverse incidents increased by 80%, and regulatory sanctions increased by 108%. Based on these statistics, the consensus is that if the agency's workload grows, lawmakers should raise its budget, not lessen its workload; otherwise, the overall quality of oversight will suffer.

Chapter 22
Medicare Billing

In November, I received several Medicare Summary Notices. A review of one revealed billing information I could not believe. These charges were for Beth from 23 January through 18 April 2019. During this period, she was in memory care and was so weak she could not turn over in bed, had difficulty getting out of her recliner without help, was using a walker or wheelchair to get around, and needed help to get dressed.

Does a person in this condition seem to be a candidate for physical therapy? The answer is no. She is an 82-year-old sick woman that will never be able to be mobile without the aid of a walker or wheelchair. Keeping this in mind, here are the services provided and billed to Medicare:

15 Physical Therapy Sessions	$1980
14 Occupation Therapy Sessions	$2310
1 Speech Therapy Session	$ 165
5 Aid/Home Health Visits	$ 400
5 Skilled Nursing Visits	$ 825
Total Billing	$6075

The period covered is for the 64 days she was in memory care. The billing states she received some therapy for 30 of those 64 days. Surprisingly, when the Medicare physical therapy payments expired, the treatment did also. The PT did not end because her mobility had improved but because Medicare stopped paying for PT services.

In addition, Medicare was billed $1225 for Home Health and Skilled Nursing even though she was in the memory care facility, so what would justify the home health and skilled nursing visit?

I realize that assisted living facilities are for-profit corporations, but getting payments of this amount for questionable services seems to be gaming the Medicare reimbursement system.

128

Chapter 23
Death Lawsuit Initiated

On 2 December, having not heard from my attorney since 5 October, a court records check revealed he had filed an Amended Complaint with the court on 8 November. My attorney had to prepare a new 19-page document duplicating the original complaint, with the only amendment being the name change from Elizabeth to me. On 9 December, the court granted the plaintiff's Motion to Amend the Complaint and gave the defendant twenty days to answer.

Legal documents typed double-spaced with a one-inch four-sided border produce many paged documents. Much of the form is a standard language used in any lawsuit document with only names and dates changed.

Section one, GENERAL ALLEGATIONS, has 8 one sentenced items.

Item 8 states, "During Elizabeth's residency at HPCC, the employees and agents under the direct control of the Defendants were negligent in the following ways." It then describes 23 one-sentence negligent items, starting with 'Failing to,' for example, "Failing to monitor and provide a safe environment for Elizabeth."

Section two, GENERAL ALLEGATIONS APPLICABLE TO DEFENDANTS, has 13 one-sentence statements comprising six pages.

One subsection reads, "Elizabeth had the following rights, and the Defendant had a duty to assure they did not violate any of the 21 one-sentence rights violations." All the rights quoted are from Florida Statute 400.022 throughout this section and other sections. My attorney quoted the 21 listed rights violations almost verbatim from the statute.

Next, the counsel lists eight one-sentence statements describing the rights violated under COUNT I, DEPRIVATION OF INFRINGEMENT OF RESIDENTS' RIGHTS. The complaint further expands this section by adding eight one-sentence acts of omission, each starting with "Failure to provide Elizabeth…." Once again, these are omissions taken from FS 400.022.

Next is COUNT II; NEGLIGENCE lists 12 one-sentence statements taken from FS 400.022 and expands upon the count by listing ten more one-sentence nursing home failures with terminology from section FS 400.022.

COUNT III, NEGLIGENCE refers to FS 400.022 and adds FS 768, the wrongful death act. This section has six one-sentence numbered items and seven claims for damages on behalf of the estate of Elizabeth. It is the only section that does not take descriptions from a statute but uses my answers to the interrogatories.

Attorneys try to impress clients with documents like the described 19-page complaint filed with the court. There is little thought on the attorney's part to compile the record. At least, in this case, it is evident that all the complaint input has either come from the client or inserted descriptions taken from the Florida statutes.

The work involved is the paralegal typing up the document, which appears to be a standard format applicable to any nursing home malpractice litigation. The double-space typing and large borders give the document quantity, the number of pages, but not necessarily quality, since my attorney inputs very little original thought.

On Christmas Eve, I had dinner with one of my golfing friends and, for,' the first time, filled another individual in on what I had been going through the last two and a half years. He could not understand how I could have gone through this experience and was amazed that I kept it all to myself. It finally felt good to share my experience with someone else.

Awaiting the next step in the litigation, I now enter the third Christmas since the lawsuit started and the first without Beth. She was like a child about Christmas. She wanted a tree to decorate the house and buy me some gifts. Her biggest regret was not being able to shop for the grandkids. She loved Christmas shopping and always expressed joy at whatever gift I bought her.

After sixty years of sharing the holidays with her, facing this one without her is hard. Even though she has been enduring constant pain during the last two Christmases, we still shared the day. This Christmas will be another day. I will play golf in the morning, feast on a deli sandwich, and watch a Netflix film. The holiday will be over, and life will go on as usual.

With the new year, I enter the third year of the lawsuit. On 3 January, not having heard from my attorney since 5 October, I accessed the court records and discovered the defendant's counsel had, on 31 December, filed a Motion to Dismiss (MTD) in answer to our amended complaint. My attorney was confident the amended complaint would make the defendant want to abate the case and go directly to arbitration.

The courts discourage MTDs because the general view is that an MTD only prolongs the litigation process. Did I mention that the defense attorney is on a retainer, so extending a case adds to his legal fees?

The document, titled "MOTION TO DISMISS and MOTION FOR MORE DEFINITE STATEMENT, AND MOTION TO STRIKE," repeats the motion to dismiss made in June 2019.

"COMES NOW, Defendants (HPCC and LMHS) by and through their undersigned counsel, and according to Rule 1.140 FRCP, now moves this court to enter an order dismissing Plaintiff's Amended Complaint and enter an order requiring the plaintiff to plead with more specificity, and to enter an order striking a portion of,' Plaintiff's Amended Complaint. The MTD then lists 23 allegations the defendant states are vague, ambiguous, and overboard that the defendant cannot reasonably frame a responsive pleading. The plaintiff should be required to plead with more specificity."

I answered the defendant's objections with more case knowledge than my attorney. I am stating the defendant's statements in summary form, removing all the legalese but presenting the jest of their complaint.

In item 2, the defendant states HPCC is a licensed Nursing Home by the state of Florida, which is owned and operated by the health system, a public health care system created by a special act of the Florida legislature. (This act includes the nursing home in the Sovereign Immunity Statute.)

I added this statement to his description, "HPCC is a facility that operates under Medicare guidelines and receives Medicare funding." (This shows the facility violated the Medicare mandates they are supposed to act under.)

In item 4, in summary, "…plaintiff alleged 'statutorily mandated residents' rights were deprived" and listed nine allegations without specifying how and when the rights violations occurred.

My answer is that the violations of rights, the embedding of a catheter, occurred for the period running from 18 May 2017, shortly after the plaintiff's admittance to the facility, and continued nonstop through 29 July 2017. At this time, the plaintiff was rushed to the emergency room. The second charged violation, dehydration, ran from 1 July 2017 until 29 July 2017, when discharged to the emergency room.

Item 5 states, "The allegations of Count I are so vague, ambiguous, and overbroad the Defendant, HPCC, cannot reasonably frame a responsive pleading."

To clear up the 'vague and ambiguous allegations', the defendant knowingly violated Medicare mandates described in CMS 20068. (Previously detailed). The catheter was not medically necessary and remained in the plaintiff for 72 days.

To further clear up the 'vague and ambiguous allegations', the nursing staff was informed by the plaintiff's representative and supported by blood tests that the plaintiff was dehydrated. When the nursing staff agreed with this diagnosis, none of the team could perform the insertion of an intravenous line to administer rehydration because of vein collapse. This inability to perform a standard medical procedure resulted in the plaintiff being rushed to the hospital in a dehydrated condition.

Item 8 is long but, in summary, states, "In paragraph 41, the plaintiff alleges the Defendants owed a duty to provide care and treatment within the standard of care, owed an obligation to provide custodial care and services consistent with resident's rights in FS 400.022, and the duty of hiring, retaining, training, supervision and firing it employees, agents, consultants, and independent contractors." (Here, the defendant referred to items in the Amended Complaint.)

In my response to paragraph 41, as detailed in item 5, it is evident that the defendant did not provide care and treatment within the standard of care.

As for paragraphs 42 and 43, I refer to CMS 20068, which states, "Has the staff involved you in care plan development, including whether interventions reflect preferences and choices and discussed the risks and benefits of a urinary catheter before insertion."

HPCC did not discuss with the plaintiff or the plaintiff's representative, nor were the chances of getting frequent urinary tract infections (UTIs) from the extended presence of an embedded catheter, the resulting kidney failure from serious UTIs, and the possibility of future fatal kidney failure.

As for paragraph 46, the defendant did not professionally train a nursing staff capable of inserting an intravenous line into the plaintiff to treat noticeable dehydration. Thus, the defendant did not meet the duty of hiring qualified nursing staff, did not train them in intravenous insertions, nor inquired whether they could perform the function.

It is also evident that the nursing staff and supervisors were not prepared to abide by Medicare mandates in CMS 20068.

In item 14, the defendant states, "Count III attempts to plead an alternative claim for wrongful death according to FS 768.16; however, fails to plead the necessary elements to state a cause of action and should therefore be dismissed."

My answer is that wrongful death is taking an individual's life resulting from the willful or negligent act/or acts of another person or persons.

According to 768.16, Florida Statutes, when a death is caused by a wrongful act (the insertion of an embedded catheter in violation of Medicare mandates), negligence (the inability of the nursing staff to perform a standard intravenous procedure), and breach of contract (resident has the right to receive adequate and proper health care and protective and support services, which, as described above the plaintiff did not receive).

Sixteen states, "Finally, Plaintiff Amended Complaint names the facility administrator as a defendant, but the complaint fails to make any allegations against the administrator."

As the facility administrator, the named defendant is responsible for the performance, or lack thereof, of all the supervisors, nursing staff, and all other employees.

Item 17 states, "Plaintiff's Complaint is based upon alleged deprivation or infringement of resident's rights, negligence and wrongful death under Chapter 400, Florida Statutes, occurring on or about 18 May 2017 to 29 July 2017."

I answer that the Plaintiff's Complaint is based on actual medical records and not on alleged deprivation or infringement of the resident's rights.

Item 21, the defendant states, "Under Section 768.28(9)(a) FS, the administrator cannot be held personally liable or named as a party defendant in this action and should be dismissed."

Here the defendant is correct. Employees of state agencies covered under the Sovereign Immunity Statute are immune from being sued. Based on this statute, the administrator should be dismissed and dropped as a named defendant. I question why the defendant did not identify this issue in their June

2019 MTD, which would have allowed the plaintiff's counsel to correct it in the amended complaint.

Not doing so in June, the defendant succeeded in prolonging the litigation by making the plaintiff's counsel issue an amended, amended complaint to remove the administrator.

The defendant did call out an issue that my attorney should have caught. The administrator, named as a defendant in our amended complaint, is an employee of the health system and is thus entitled to the provisions of the Florida Waiver of Sovereign Immunity Act.

The act states, "No officer, employee, or agent of the state shall be held personally liable in tort as named as a party defendant in action for injury or damage suffered as a result of any act, event, or an omission of action in the scope of his employment or function."

Although the complaint does not make any allegations against the administrator, he is always material to criticism since he was an employee of the health system. As per Florida Statutes, he cannot be held personally liable or named a party defendant in this action and should be dismissed. Based on the defendant's claim, I emailed my counsel on 5 January.

From my review of court records, your belief that the defendant would want to abate the action and move to arbitration after receiving the amended complaint was dreaming. I elected to answer the defendant's MTD and will furnish you with my answers upon request. Since the administrator cannot be named in the complaint, is answering the MTD a moot issue? Will a new amended complaint have to be issued?

On 14 January, I resend the e-mail with the subject line 'Rule Regulating the Florida Bar, Chapter 4', Rule 4-1.4. This rule states the following:

Rule 4-1.4 COMMUNICATION

Informing the Client of the Status of Representation, a lawyer shall: Promptly inform the client of any decision or circumstance for which these rules require the client's informed consent. Consult with the client about how the client's objectives are accomplished. Keep the client reasonably informed about the status of the matter. Promptly comply with reasonable requests for information.

Duty to Explain Matters to Client: A lawyer shall explain a matter to the extent necessary to allow the client to make informed decisions about the representation. Communication between the lawyer and client is essential for the client to participate in the presentation effectively.

A lawyer's regular contact with clients will minimize the occasions a client will need to request information concerning the representation. When a client makes a reasonable request for information, it requires prompt compliance with the request, or if a quick response is not possible, that the lawyer, or a member of the lawyer's staff, acknowledge receipt of the request and advise the client when they may expect a reply.

Rule 4-1.3 DILIGENCE

A lawyer shall act with reasonable diligence and promptness in representing a client. A lawyer must control his workload so he can handle each matter competently.

As documented throughout this story, it is obvious my counsel still needs to meet the requirement of Chapter 4 as described above, but I need help changing counsel mid-case. I even explored the idea of representing myself. I have a law degree obtained in the 1960s before the invention of the word processor and the internet. After reading a story about Clarence Darrow, the attorney in the Scopes Monkey trial, I decided I would like to have a law degree, not to practice, but to say I had a law degree.

Seeing an ad for getting a degree through mail-order study, I contacted the school, paid the $400 enrollment fee, a considerable sum in the 60s, and became a student. I received a 36-volume law library to study for written essay tests administered after reading each chapter. The question answers were typed and sent to the school for grading. I did all my studying at night, and after seven years of study, I finally obtained my law degree in February 1968.

Using my law knowledge and internet research, I have often managed to piss off my attorney by asking him questions a typical client would not ask. A prime example is trying to hold him to the Rules Regulating the Florida Bar described above. However, not being licensed in Florida, the idea of representing myself is a moot point.

I got an answer, and we finally established some dialog for the first time in two years.

Attorney: You seem to be one of those 'forests for the trees' kind of people.

Me: Probably an accurate description of me, but humor me. Suppose the Sovereign Immunity Act covers the administrator, making him immune from litigation, as claimed in the defendants' latest MTD. Why wasn't this fact covered in their MTD filed in June? Do you have to file another amended complaint to remove him, or can you acknowledge their contention in the MTD response?

Attorney: Thank you for also humoring me. We can fight him on not including the administrator in the earlier MTD, or we could fight to keep him in; however, I see a potential stipulation between the parties to agree to amend again without hearing, take the administrator out and get an answer to the complaint from opposing counsel.

Me: Thanks; this is the kind of information that will allow me to see beyond the trees. Continued tree clearing and updated case information will let me see the forest.

His response was, "I like this."

Chapter 24
2nd Amended Complaint

Much of the legalization you read here may have been read previously and repeated because it is used in different documents to respond to the defense attorney's questions. In other motions, the defense will ask the same question in diverse ways, but in most cases, my response will be the same as in his earlier actions. These court records are presented in lengthy legalize to show the reader why lawsuits take years to litigate.

On 18 January, I got the first billing from the probate attorney. Though the case is still in litigation, with no sign of ending, I still must start paying for the probate filing. I was billed $1,306 for the first installment of the $3,000 fees.

On 27 January, my counsel prepared a new, 20-page SECOND AMENDED COMPLIANT AND DEMAND FOR JURY TRIAL. It duplicates, except for two added items addressing the nursing home administrator, the 'AMENDED COMPLAINT' filed on 9 December 2019.

The new Complaint calls out by name the administrator stating, "That at all times material hereto, the defendant, was licensed by the State of Florida and was serving as the administrator during Elizabeth's residency. According to Florida Statutes, the defendant bears liability arising from his official capacity."

I don't understand this change since the defendant's MTD filed on 3 December stated that "Accordingly, under Section 768.28 Florida Statutes, the administrator cannot be held personally liable or named as a party defendant in this action, and the administrator should be dropped as a named defendant."

How his now being named in more detail in the new motion changes the fact of him being immune is beyond my comprehension. Only a liberal interpretation of the statute may make him a defendant.

Addressing MTD's claim, the Amended Complaint does not make any allegations against the administrator.

According to Florida Statutes, the MTD claims that based on the statement starting with 'No officer and ending with his employment or function,'' the administrator is immune from litigation.

However, the MTD did not continue that quoted sentence, "unless such officer, employee, or agent acted in bad faith or with malicious purpose or exhibiting wanton and willful disregard of human rights, safety, or property." The plaintiff could argue that the administrator handled the actions of his nursing supervisor and staff who committed the 'willful disregard of human rights'; however, even using this liberal interpretation of 768.28 (9), why is it necessary to include him?

He responded, "I am continuing to discuss the amendment with opposing counsel." I read this to mean he will not submit the Second Amendment Complaint to the court until opposing counsel agrees to include the administrator, even though the defendant stated he is opposed to naming him.

Checking court records to see the results of the 10 February meeting revealed the following notation made by the judge.

"The Court decided to proceed after waiting approximately 10 minutes, and Plaintiff's attorney still did not appear. Motion granted with leave to amend." Having known about this scheduled Court meeting for weeks, I thought my attorney insulted the court by failing to appear. The court granted the defendant's Motion to Dismiss.

My attorney pissed me off by being a no-show, and I again contacted the attorney I had discussed firing my counsel. He repeated the improbability of finding an attorney to take over an existing sovereign immunity case. Prosecuting a lawsuit against a state agency covered by sovereign immunity is expensive and time-consuming. The state agencies will make it a point to slow-walk the case since their attorney is on a retainer and time is money and run the costs to the plaintiff higher with time.

The Florida legislature and the medical lobby have done an excellent job of preventing someone suffering from a malpractice injury from suing a hospital or nursing home designated a state agency. Thus, due to medical malpractice or negligence, many injured parties cannot find counsel to represent them and suffer the effects of such malpractice without redress. The prime objective of the legislation was to make suing a state agency so tricky that, through the setting of caps, the state would eliminate many valid lawsuits. I cannot change attorney.

Having waited one week to get a response from my attorney detailing his no-show reasoning, I sent him an e-mail asking him: Now that you have pissed off the judge, when do you expect to answer the defendant's MTD? I was surprised to get an answer and find out I now have a new attorney, my third.

I return to something I read: "Not all so-called law practices practice law and will accept lawsuits with the hope they will be able to figure the case out eventually." At times, I wonder whether I retained one. My first contact with my new attorney convinced me that I finally got an attorney.

On 18 February, I received a professionally written answer to my question addressed to attorney two. He informed me that the leave to amend means my attorney must include more specific facts in the Amended Complaint. A new complaint filed with the Court on 17 February addressed these issues. My attorney said the Complaint is vague to protect my claim. Before the formal discovery process, a complaint is filed where the plaintiff will learn more about the defendant's view of the case.

My problem is that the Second Amended Complaint is still naming the administrator as a defendant, and by doing so, I would expect opposing counsel to file another MTD. The defense did file another MTD on 26 February, with issues almost duplicating those detailed in their 31 December MTD.

On 1/8/2020, I reached my 87th birthday. My goal is to outlive the lawsuit, and the purpose of the defendant's attorney is to drag the case out to see if he can counter my goal.

My attorney answered my question about how he would treat this new MTD. We will tweak a few things on the Complaint but fight them on the rest. They have yet to reach out for hearing dates, but you will see a responsive motion with an amended complaint and opposition to several points of their action.

"This should be the last round, and I expect a successful hearing." I do not understand what he just wrote; at least he is responsive to my questions. I answered all the defendant's complaints and sent them to him.

The plaintiff's response in opposition to the defendant's MTD complaint states.

The plaintiff's claim that HPCC violated Medicare-mandated directives (CMS 20068) for indwelling catheters. It failed to have nurses who could perform the functions required to insert an intravenous line, detailing the violations claimed. The plaintiff has shown that HPCC was negligent in fulfilling its statutes to provide the reasonable care standard to the plaintiff.

There should be no requirement for a specific time and place for the negligence acts since they continued from the plaintiff's entry to the facility to her eviction 72 days later. The plaintiff has alleged sufficient facts to give the defendant "fair notice of the nature of the claim and the grounds upon which they rest."

The Court, considering an MTD, must accept that the facts alleged in the Complaint are actual. The Court considering an MTD may dismiss the case only if it decides the plaintiff can prove 'no set of facts supporting their claim. The plaintiff has met the burden of presenting a 'set of facts.'

Defendant's 26 February MTD has the same 27 objections stated in their 31 December MTD, which I answered the same as detailed previously. The present MTD should be denied.

Despite the defense's rejection of the plaintiff naming the administrator as a defendant, my attorney seems determined to have him remain in the suit. In the MTD, the defense states that the plaintiff: "Fails to make any allegations against the administrator" and fails to recognize under the Florida Statutes, "No officer shall be named as a party defendant in any action in the scope of their employment function."

Thus the administrator should be dropped as a named defendant. I, the novice lawyer, must agree with the defendant. We should drop the administrator. Continuing to name him as a defendant will generate more defendant MTDs. The only section of the statute that would make the administrator liable states, "Unless such officer acted in bad faith or with malicious purpose or in a manner exhibiting wanton and willful disregard of human rights, safety or property." The administrator exhibited none of such behavior.

My attorney mentioned he had conferred with opposing counsel to resolve the issues raised in the MTD. Rule 3.01 requires the moving party, the defendant, to consult with counsel for the opposing party in a reasonable faith effort to resolve the issues raised by the motion. They solved none of the problems.

His response was to thank me for my MTD response, but the idea was to be successful at the hearing. We must evaluate their contentions and amend what we may not prevail at the hearing but file a response to what we will prevail on. The administrator being listed as a defendant is a prime example of something we will fight at the hearing. We need to avoid another MTD because we intend on having a hearing on the current MTD as it is ripe to be heard.

When I asked for an interpretation of the 'is ripe' comment, he responded that it is grown because the opposing counsel has finally shown all his cards about his legal objections to the Complaint. Now we can address it without concern for another MTD following it. He again mentions that some of the changes will require an amended complaint. He also said he would be responding to the whole MTD, and the judge would have a copy in advance to consider and review at the hearing.

It is the defense's responsibility to schedule oral arguments with the court after an MTD is filed, and, as per my attorney, they have not filed to get on the judge's Motion Calendar. There is no timeline for when the defense must file to get on the calendar. My response was that if there is no timeline in which he must file, what incentive does the defendant have to get on the calendar? He responded that if the defendant thought their MTD would be successful, that would be their incentive. The plaintiff's hands are tied until the opposing counsel decides.

I prepared a newspaper op-ed seeking to bring this case out of the dark halls of justice and into the light of day. Exposure may be the incentive the defendant needs to move the case along. I composed an op-ed for submittal to the local newspaper, putting my frustration before the public. I would write it to satisfy my frustration but wait to submit it until I ran it by my attorney.

I asked him if I was bound by any gag order that would keep me from going public about the lawsuit. He answered that any gag order did not bind me, but he would advise against it because it may compromise further negotiations. I took his advice for now.

COVID-19 entered the picture in March and could delay the case ending indefinitely. With the closing of the courts, the lawsuit has come to an unforeseeable halt. Even when courts open and progress on the suit should continue, the defendant could go from a slow walk in processing the case to a crawl. As mentioned, being an eighty-seven-year-old highly susceptible to contracting the virus, the defendant can stall the proceedings with the possibility of my contacting the virus and possible death.

Chapter 25
3rd Amended Complaint

On 6 April, my attorney submitted a 26-page MOTION TO AMEND COMPLAINT AND RESPONSE TO MOTION FOR MORE DEFINITE STATEMENT in answer to the defendant's 26 February MTD.

It states, "The motion is in response to the defendant's MTD by filing a Third Amended Complaint following the Fla. R. Civ. P.1.190 and as good grounds states: Rule 1.190 Florida Rules of Civil Procedure, provides a party may amend a pleading with leave of court" and "Leave of court shall be given freely when justice so requires."

Plaintiff has tried in good faith to engage with the Defendants with a complaint that could be stipulated, and the Defendants have not responded to the plaintiff's multiple requests. The Third Amended Complaint shall be responsive to Defendant's Motion for a More Definite Statement.

WHEREFORE, the plaintiff prays this Honorable Court Grant an Order giving leave to the plaintiff to file the attached Complaint and any other relief this Honorable Court considers just and fair.

I noticed in the new Complaint that my counsel still names the administrator as a defendant, and the statute is specific. Even with the defendant's counsel making it an issue in their MTD, my counsel still insists on naming the administrator as a co-defendant.

The amended Complaint is titled THIRD AMENDED COMPLAINT AND DEMAND FOR JURY TRIAL. It lists 11 items and concludes with item 12, which states. Under Sections 768.28 and 400.0233, Florida Statutes, all conditions precedent to the filing of this action have been satisfied or fulfilled.

Item 13 is entitled CERTIFICATE OF COUNSEL, which is the defining statement of the Complaint and the suit and states: Under Florida Statutes, Section 400.0233, the undersigned attorney of record does now certify he conducted a reasonable investigation as to the matters alleged herein and determined that there are grounds for a good faith belief that the care and treatment were negligent of Elizabeth and that grounds exist for the filing of this action against the defendant.

The following GENERAL ALLEGATIONS APPLICABLE TO DEFENDANTS. It mirrors the allegations described in the Second Amended Complaint, with many item descriptions expanded upon and some significant changes. The first is item 19. Let me digress. If you recall, one of the crucial acts of misconduct was HPCC's use of an embedded catheter, disregarding Medicare's CMS 20068 mandates on the use of a catheter. Items 19 and 20 refute the defendant's defense that the catheter was medically required.

Item 19 states: To justify the urinary catheter being necessary for reasons other than employee convenience, HPCC entered into Elizabeth's plan of care that she had been diagnosed with obstructive uropathy, i.e., a urinary blockage. However, item 20 contradicts this and states: Yet there is no mention in any of Elizabeth's other medical records showing a diagnosis of obstructive uropathy. HPCC is trying to justify its procedures using false information.

Item 22, also new to this amendment, states: Due to the use of this urinary catheter, not for treatment of any medical condition but simply for the convenience of agents and employees of HPCC, Elizabeth contracted a series of urinary tract infections requiring added hospitalization due to antibiotic resistance.

Added item 23 states: In addition, while a resident of HPCC, on or about July 12th, 2017, Elizabeth was discovered on the floor, next to her wheelchair, the agents and employees of HPCC having allowed her to fall unwitnessed, despite being on notice Elizabeth presented a significant fall risk. This item adds another example of HPCC's failure to provide the contracted care in HPCC's procedure manual.

Two other items dealt with the dehydration episode she experienced at HPCC. Item 26 states:

When asked by Plaintiff John whether Elizabeth's dry condition might require admission to an emergency room, agents and employees of HPCC actively dissuaded him from seeking emergency room treatment. Item 27 states: Despite eventually inserting an intravenous tube into Elizabeth to rehydrate her, her condition had become such that emergency room treatment for dehydration was necessary.

As an example of the difference in professionalism between my new and old attorneys, I would like to show an item description from each addressing the same subject.

Old description: According to Fla. Stat. 400.022, Elizabeth had the following rights: the Defendants had a duty to ensure they did not violate them.

New description: Under Section 400.022, Florida Statutes, the state and federal rules and regulations adopted and promulgated thereunder according to 400.022(1)(I), all of which constitute a part of the established and recognized healthcare standards within the community, Elizabeth had the following rights. Defendants had a duty to ensure they did not violate the following rights.

The updated version expands the descriptions of those rights detailed in the Second Amended Complaint.

The substantial change from the Second Amended Complaint is with Count III, entitled NEGLIGENCE. It now reads in the Third Amended Complaint as Count III WRONGFUL DEATH: The Defendants' negligence in ordering a catheter for nonexistent obstructive uropathy—solely for the convenience of agents and employees of the defendant—as well as the defendant's failure to effectively prevent and treat the urinary tract infections caused by this unnecessary catheterization, directly and proximately caused the death of Elizabeth. The first time my attorney identified a negligent act by HPCC as the cause of Elizabeth's death.

On 13 April, the MTD hearing was held by telephone conference due to COVID-19 not allowing face-to-face contact. The judge granted the defendant's MTD without prejudice (in part) to address the issues on the negligence counts and the wrongful death issues. The judge also granted with prejudice as to the administrator individually, and the court granted the plaintiff thirty days to amend the Complaint.

However, even though the court has removed the administrator from the Complaint, my attorney insists on leaving him therein. His doing so started the following series of e-mails.

Question: Why is the administrator still named a co-defendant when agency employees are immune from being called a defendant in a lawsuit?

Answer: Under the Sovereign Immunity Statute, he can be named a defendant in a lawsuit in his 'official capacity.' As you know from the minutes, it is one of the issues challenged. He can be named as per Fla. Stat. 768.28(9)(a) "The exclusive remedy for injury or damage suffered as a result of an act, event, or omission of an officer, employee, or agent of the state or any of its subdivision or constitutional officers shall be action against the head of such entity in her or his official capacity…."

Question: The remainder of that sentence reads, "Unless such act or omission was committed in bad faith or with malicious purpose or in a manner showing wanton and willful disregard of human rights, safety, or property." It would take a very liberal interpretation of that sentence to imply that the administrator's actions, or lack thereof, meet those criteria. Since the administrator would not be liable for damages, what is accomplished by naming him a co-defendant?

Answer: The exception you include allows the official to be sued in their capacity if they are malicious, as that is outside the scope of their power.

Question: How would you define malicious?

Answer: Malicious refers to malic, a state of mind that accompanies the intentional doing or a wrongful act without justification or excuse.

Question: Humor me. A sovereign can be sued in court, but only for prospective injunction relief to prevent further violations, and the administrator does not meet this condition. As for malicious conduct, in a case just last year, the court interpreted 'Malicious purpose' as conduct committed with spite, ill will, and hate, an extremely high bar to hurdle. Why wouldn't a defense attorney use either of the above objections in an MTD disputing the naming of the administrator?

Answer: Good question. I am still trying to figure out what the defense attorney is thinking. Drafting the changes per the judge will take little time, but I found out before the hearing that the defense attorney has some issues with the new Complaint. I have already drafted a response to anticipation issues. What will take time is getting with him. I want to get this case moving.

Question: I appreciate working with you, mainly the two-way exchange of information, so do not get upset with my trying to play lawyer. I have a good rapport with my new counsel but need help getting him off the need to name the administrator as a co-defendant.

Curious, I looked up the legal definition of a motion granted 'with and without prejudice.' A motion granted 'with prejudice' means it is permanently dismissed. In contrast, a motion dismissed 'without prejudice' means the plaintiff can try and fix the problems the defendant identified in the MTD. The court allows the plaintiff to correct the defects and refile the Complaint on its merits.

The judge has also 'with prejudice' removed the administrator from the Complaint as a co-defendant.

Let me review where we are now in the lawsuit. The court must approve the Third Amendment before issuing it. In addition, it is now a new complaint with the administrator removed as a named defendant. The defendant will have ten days to respond to the new Complaint and may issue another MTD, and we will be right back to where we were in June 2018.

My e-mail chain with my attorney about including the administrator in the Complaint was an exercise in futility. The judge settled that issue by stating, "Motion is granted 'with prejudice' as to the administrator individually." He eliminated naming the administrator as a co-defendant in the lawsuit, an issue I had raised since my attorney issued the first complaint in April 2019.

A novice with a law degree obtained in 1968 should not be advising my attorney, who will get 40% of any settlement. The Florida Sovereign Immunity Statutes make an officer of a sovereign immunity agency immune from being named a defendant in a lawsuit. It took a judge to tell my attorney the same facts I had been preaching for over a year. The episode that pisses me off is that we had just spent days exchanging e-mails where I told him the administrator is immune.

He continued to tell me how he would find exceptions, allowing him to include him in a new complaint, even though he knew the judge had made the issue moot. We are now back to where we were in April 2019. My attorney has 30 days to issue a new Amended Complaint, and the defendant will have 20 days to respond. Think of all the unnecessary motions and amendments filed addressing the naming of the administrator as a defendant. After a rereading, I sent the following e-mail to my attorney.

Reading the minutes of the 13 April hearing prompted me to find the legal definition of 'with and without prejudice.' Based on those interpretations, our e-mail chain over the past week was just an exercise in futility. Correct me if I am wrong, but I interpret the statement 'Motion granted with prejudice' as to the administrator individually means the administrator has been permanently removed from the Complaint as a co-defendant.

You knew this fact, so why did we waste our time last week trying to find a way to include him in the suit? I informed LGF in 2019 that the administrator did not meet the criteria necessary to be named a defendant in the lawsuit and should be removed. It took a judge to tell you the same facts I had been telling you for over a year. I am still waiting for a response to my e-mail.

The judge issued the following order on 17 April in response to the April 13th meeting. This matter came before the court on 13 April 2020 for a hearing on Defendant's Motion to Dismiss, Motion to Strike, and Motion for a More Definite Statement. The court, being fully advised on the premises, orders as follows:

Defendant's Motion to Dismiss Counts I, II, and III of Plaintiff's Second Amended Complaint is now granted without prejudice. Paragraphs 41, 42, 44–49, and 51 are now stricken; Defendant (the administrator's name) is dismissed as a named party defendant with prejudice. The plaintiff shall have thirty (30) days from the date of this order to file a Third Amended Complaint.

On 28 April, my attorney submitted a 26-page THIRD AMENDED COMPLAINT to the court, revising the Complaint sent to the court on 9 April. The Complaint was sent for review but has yet to be submitted for action. This new Complaint consists of only 12 pages versus the previous 26, eliminating the administrator from the suit.

The most significant and professionally described change is in the section entitled GENERAL ALLEGATIONS APPLICABLE TO DEFENDANTS, which lists 27 allegations of malicious conduct. Removal of the administrator has resulted in reducing four pages from the Complaint.

The following change is in the section entitled COUNT I, DEPRIVATION OR INFRINGEMENT OF RESIDENT'S RIGHTS.

Item 34 of this section states: "The acts and omissions of the Defendant which deprived Elizabeth of her resident rights include, but are not limited to." The 9 April revision listed 24 acts and omissions. The new amended Complaint has reduced this number to 7 actions and omissions by presenting only the most relevant acts, thus reducing the defendant's attorney's nitpicking of the listing and reducing the Amended Complaint by five more pages. You wonder how my new attorney can state the same facts in 5 fewer pages. It again leads me to believe my past attorneys worked on the theory of quantity, namely the number of pages, equal quality.

The section COUNT II NEGLIGENCE extended the description to read BREACH OF STANDARD CARE. The paragraphs ordered stricken by the judge have been removed, thus reducing the Complaint by another six pages. The section still makes the same breach of standard care but in fewer words.

The new Complaint entitled COUNT III NEGLIGENT HIRING added a section. The first four items in this section detail the defendants' duty to hire, train, and supervise employees to ensure they deliver care and services to residents safely and beneficially. Item 47 states that the defendants breached the duties owed to Elizabeth by not hiring, training, and supervising employees so that such employees deliver the above-described services.

The count summarized item 48 to read: "As a direct and proximate cause of the Defendant's acts and omissions in breaching their duties, Elizabeth suffered bodily injury and resulting pain and suffering, disability, disfigurement, mental anguish, loss of capacity for the enjoyment of life, expense of hospitalization, medical and nursing care, and treatment, and aggravation of a previously existing condition," a standard sentence inserted in every medical malpractice suit with only the name of the plaintiff changed.

The concluding section is COUNT IV-WRONGFUL DEATH. It again reviews the acts and omissions of the defendant. It concludes with the statement: "WHEREFORE, the plaintiff, as personal representative of the estate of Elizabeth, demands all damages which he is entitled to recover under the Florida Wrongful Death Act, including loss of future support, income, companionship, care, comfort, society and for mental pain and suffering from the date of injury to Elizabeth and into the future, with costs against Defendant HPCC, and a trial by jury."

On 5 May, the defendant answered the Third Amended Complaint with a 9-page response. To summarize the response, they agreed that Elizabeth was a resident of HPCC. HPCC was legally mandated to provide her with nursing home residents' rights under FS 400.022. Still, the defendant denied every other allegation described in the 12 pages of the amended Complaint. They listed all of the allegation identification numbers and rejected each by number. The defendant did not acknowledge being responsible for any of the 54 allegations.

In addition, the defendant added three pages to the ANSWER TO PLAINTIFF'S THIRD AMENDED COMPLAINT with what they refer to as SEVENTEEN AFFIRMATIVE DEFENSES. I will not list all seventeen defenses, but one can only understand this document's complexity and legal jargon if one can see it. I have tried to respond to only the defenses that apply to the case. The defense will cite every reason he can think of that could be used, knowing many would not be used, but it is better to list them and not need them than to need them and not list them.

Defendants have specifically answered each paragraph of the Third Amended Complaint, now claiming different and affirmative defenses.

THIRD AFFIRMATIVE DEFENSE: Defendants assert the incident or damages complained of by plaintiffs were caused by the condition and independent intervening acts beyond the Defendants' control. So, the Plaintiffs are precluded from recovery for the alleged damages.

How the defense can claim this as a defense is beyond my comprehension. The reason is arguing that the insertion of an indwelling catheter, in a flagrant violation of Medicare mandates, and the failure of the nursing staff to be able to insert an intravenous feeding line were beyond the defendant's control. If not, who was it?

FOURTH AFFIRMATIVE DEFENSE: Defendants are entitled to the applicable provision of Florida Statutes 766.102, 766.104, 768.13, 768.28, 768.76, 768.78.

This defense necessitated my looking up all the referred-to statutes on the internet and finding a significant one that may be applicable.

766.102 "Medical negligence, standards or recovery; expert witness." It states: (1) In any action for recovery of damages based on the death or personal injury of any person in which it is alleged that such death or injury resulted from the negligence of a health care provider, the claimant shall have the burden of proving by the greater weight of evidence that the alleged action of the health care provider represented a breach of the prevailing professional standard of care for the health care provider.

"The general professional standard of care for a given health provider shall be the level of care, skill, and treatment which, in light of all relevant surrounding circumstances, is recognized as acceptable and appropriate by reasonably prudent similar health care providers," failure to follow Medicare mandates on the use of a catheter is a breach of the prevailing professional standard of care meeting the medical negligence standard.

FOURTEENTH AFFIRMATIVE DEFENSE: That such injury as a plaintiff may have suffered was solely the result of the natural and inevitable process of human disease and condition of recognized therapy risks to treat the same. I included this to show how far the defendant will go to say they were not at fault.

FIFTEENTH AFFIRMATIVE DEFENSE: The medical intervention was undertaken with the patient's informed consent compliance with Fla. Stat. 766.103.

766.103 Florida Medical Consent Law, in summary, this statute states: "Obtaining the patient's consent or another person authorized to permit the patient" was following an acceptable standard of medical practice. The individual giving the consent would generally understand the procedure, the medically acceptable alternative methods or treatments, and the inherent risks and hazards in the proposed treatment or process. Approval in writing meets the requirements; the plaintiff gave no such consent.

I have summarized some of the 99 documents submitted to the court to propel the lawsuit's journey through the halls of justice. As the reader will see, it is not a straight line, and it is like going from Boston to New York via way of Chicago, to use an analogy. The frustrating element of this lawsuit is that all this documentation is needed to take a case to trial when both the defendant and plaintiff's attorneys know the case will never see the inside of a courtroom.

The case could have been settled quickly by the two parties entering into mediation and coming to a settlement agreement. Certain aspects of this lawsuit are against a quick settlement.

The defendant, with deep pockets, has retained outside counsel to prosecute the case at an estimated $50 to $250 per billable hour. To settle this case without the defense going through Chicago would kill the golden goose laying the golden egg for the defendant's counsel. In addition, the trip through Chicago requires the plaintiff's attorney, compensated by a 40% contingency fee of the settlement, to travel the same route.

This journey also makes the plaintiff's counsel think twice about taking a sovereign immunity lawsuit. The plaintiff's counsel could spend the same amount of time on a two hundred-million-dollar case with a 40% fee as he will on a two hundred-thousand-dollar lawsuit that will pay a 40% contingency fee. So, why should the defense counsel settle a case in three months when he can take three years to accomplish the same results?

After months of Complaints, Amended Complaints, Second Complaints, Motions to Dismiss, and numerous other documents, my attorney finally submitted the Third Amended Complaint to the court.

Chapter 26
Discovery

The legal definition of 'discovery' is a procedural device employed by a party to a civil action before trial, requiring the adverse party to show information essential for preparing the requesting party's case that the other party knows or has.

The term 'civil law' primarily concerns the failure of one party to do something or avoid doing something that causes harm to another person. In civil lawsuits, the plaintiff has the burden of proof, called "preponderance of the evidence, which refers to the weight of the evidence, not the amount."

A plaintiff does not have to prove a wrongful death civil case beyond a reasonable doubt; they must convince a judge that the nursing home's maleficence caused the plaintiff's death. Civil damages, such as would be awarded in this case, are monetary awards granted when a person suffers a loss due to another party's wrongful or negligent actions.

Even though the defendant has denied all the allegations made in the Third Amended Complaint as detailed above, they have now issued a NOTICE OF SERVING INTERROGATORIES which states: The defendant propounds interrogatories to the plaintiff, to be responded to within the time and manner prescribed by Florida Rules of Civil Procedure. Attached to this is DEFENDANT'S INTERROGATORIES TO PLAINTIFF. The questions in this section are addressed to me to answer.

Interrogatories are written questions submitted by the defendant and must be answered by the plaintiff. The defendant may submit up to 25 questions which must be answered by a minimum one-sentence extended response. The law states that the plaintiff and defendant should exchange information about the facts of the underlying incident, the plaintiff's allegations, and the defendant's potential response.

I realize discovery is a part of the legal system, but I question whether it is another procedure that will delay a suit settlement. Support for this contention is evident in some of the following 15 questions the defense asks me to answer. I question the relevancy of the following questions with the defendant's counsel, knowing that for me to answer them would take weeks of research. Most of these questions have been answered previously in interrogatories, but the defense has the right to ask again.

Q: Give a full description, including inclusive dates, of each injury and illness of the decedent during the ten (10) years preceding their death.

Q: The name and address of each physician consulted by the decedent concerning their health, specifying the purpose for which the physician was consulted for each occasion.

Q: What is the name and address of each hospital where the decedent was a patient preceding their death, specifying inclusive dates of hospitalization?

Q: Itemize all medical and hospital expenses incurred or paid because of the death of your decedent, the date each fee was incurred, the name and address of the person to whom each of such costs was paid or incurred, and the dates of payments.

The last four questions on the interrogatories were the relevant ones.

Q: If you contend that your decedent suffered conscious physical pain or mental anguish, please state the following: the exact time on the day of the accident at which the accident occurred; the same time after that to which they died; the exact period they consciously survived the accident; the actual period between the time of the accident and the time of their death during which they suffered conscious physical pain and mental anguish.

A: The incidents contributing to Elizabeth's death started shortly after her admittance to HPCC on 18 May 2017 and continued to escalate until she left HPCC on 29 July 2017. As a result of the medical misconduct of HPCC, she continued to suffer severe urinary tract infections, many resulting in trips to the emergency room and admittance to the hospital. She suffered increasingly severe painful urinary tract infections and depression from 18 May 2017 to 8 July 2019, when she died in hospice from kidney failure brought on by the continued urinary tract infections.

Q: State the name and address of each person known or believed by you, your attorney, or other representatives to be: an eye witness to the occurrence described in the Complaint, and state his location at such time; not an eye witness, but who has or may have knowledge of the facts upon which the allegations of negligence are based.

A: The eyewitnesses to the malfeasance were the plaintiff and the agents and employees of the defendant. They were aware of and did not have the staff experience to correct the apparent deterioration of Elizabeth. The most informative eyewitness is the plaintiff, who saw all acts of omission and commission detailed.

Q: Describe each act or omission of the defendant you contend constituted negligence contributing to the legal cause of the incident.

A: The case is based not only on acts of omission but also on acts of commission. HPCC, a Medicare facility in direct violation of Medicare mandates, embedded a urinary catheter for no known medical necessity, knowing that they would be subjecting Elizabeth to a lifetime of urinary tract infections. As for an act or omission, the facility admitting Elizabeth was severely dehydrated did not have a staff nurse who could perform the insertion of an intravenous line.

As stated, the defendant and the plaintiff can question each other using interrogatories. Based on that right, my attorney issued to the court and defendant PLAINTIFF'S NOTICE OF SERVING FIRST SET OF NURSING HOME INTERROGATORES to answer the attached interrogatories.

On 20 May, I had a 75-minute phone conference with my attorney, which was informative and beneficial to both of us to speak and get to know each other. My first order of business had to do with my not being notified that the defendant had answered the Third Amended Complaint and finding out the defendant had responded to it only by my accessing the Court records.

I told him the Third Amended Complaint was an excellent, professionally prepared complaint that concisely summarized our allegations, reducing the Complaint by 26 to 12 pages. I was particularly upset about not knowing the defendant's affirmative defenses. He told me the dismissal of all allegations detailed in the Complaint was expected, and the listed affirmative defenses are used in every defendant's answer to a Complaint. He stated he would send future copies of the court-submitted document.

We then discussed the affirmative defenses. After reading the statutes the defense's affirmatives referred to, I questioned why he included some of them. He told me they had no intention of using all of them, but the defense wanted a variety of referred-to statutes so he could use them, not all of them.

Here I learned something. I believed a nursing home under sovereign immunity could not go to trial, but damages would be assessed in arbitration. Let me here review the events of pre-suit mediation. After unsuccessful conciliation in March 2019, I asked attorney number two if the next step was to go to trial. He informed me that the nursing home contract stated that all disputes with the nursing home would be settled through arbitration.

Based on his information, I prepared the previously detailed arbitration presentation. When I told my present attorney of my understanding that the nursing home must go to arbitration rather than trial as per attorney two, he assured me my belief was invalid. HPCC can go to trial but would not want to because of the bad publicity it would generate. Now I know why attorney number two never answered my e-mails asking when he would request arbitration after being informed of an arbitration clause; a nursing home contract review found no such agreement.

The contract states, "The parties expressly consent to and agree to the venue for any legal action as being solely the Twentieth Judicial Circuit, regardless of any laws affecting venue." After my conference, I am sure, as mentioned before, that my two previous attorneys were not competent to handle a sovereign immunity case. The firm took the case with the idea that they could learn while processing. My present counsel, who has been with the firm briefly, was given my case based on experience with similar issues. My research on arbitration, especially my presentation, will still be usable for a jury presentation.

After our discussion, the conference went well, and I have a higher opinion of my counsel's ability. He has agreed to keep me updated as the case progresses, and I can schedule a conference whenever I need to talk to him. I told him I have a law degree and may ask him questions that 99% of his clients would not ask, so humor me when I ask them.

Should you tell your attorney that you also have a law degree? It is something like telling your doctor you have a WebMD degree and am now going to ask him medical questions obtained from the internet. Overall, the conference cleared the air, and I am confident of my attorney's ability to prosecute this case.

The defendant had their shot at us to answer their interrogatories; now it is our turn. My attorney has submitted a document titled PLAINTIFF'S FIRST REQUEST TO PRODUCE TO DEFENDANT to the court and the defendant.

A request for the production of documents, a process presented during discovery, is a request made by a party to civil litigation for the opposing party to submit certain documents, in this case, to the plaintiff for his inspection. The 'discovery' rules govern what evidence is subject to examination by the plaintiff.

Any non-privileged matter relevant to either party's claim or defense is discoverable through a request to produce documents. The receiving party may grant or deny the requesting party the right to inspect the identified records. A request for production allows each party to collect and organize their respective evidence in preparation for trial. During discovery, anything not privileged about the case is generally discoverable. A request to produce documents will be comprehensive in identifying the records requested. The document reads:

According to Rule 1.350, Florida Rules of Civil Procedure request the Defendants to produce or copy the documents for inspection. The next item in the paper is called 'Definitions.' It then defines the word 'documents,' with a three-paragraph definition of what the plaintiff means by documents, followed by much legalese before getting to the heart of the request. The defendant has 45 days to respond to the demand for production.

DEFENDANT SHALL PRODUCE THE FOLLOWING ITEMS AND MATTERS. This section asks 65 comprehensive questions or requests for documents such as facility policies. All 65 requests for information are valid, but it may take the defendant 45 days to document the requested information. I will not list the items ordered in the 12-page document but will wait for the defendant's response and update you at that time.

My attorney submitted to the court a document titled PLAINTIFF'S NOTICE OF SERVING FIRST SET OF NURSING HOME INTERROGATORIES. The paper responded to the defendant serving the earlier detailed interrogatories to me.

Here the plaintiff has submitted to the defendant 22 questions to be answered by the nursing home and the administrator within 30 days after receipt. The questions were much more explicate, asking for detailed responses that would give the plaintiff a good picture of the HPCCs defense. Two pertinent questions were:

Do you claim that any health care provider, including but not limited to physicians who attend to the plaintiff, fell below any accepted standard of care in their treatment?

Do you claim that any physician attending to the plaintiff while a patient at HPCC issued any inappropriate, incorrect, or substandard order for medication or other treatment?

You can see why getting an attorney to take a sovereign immunity case is so difficult for the contingency cap placed on the attorney. At this point in the process, the plaintiff and defendant's attorneys have submitted 53 documents to the court encompassing 271 pages, and the case may be months or years away from being settled.

For every paper the defense produces, the plaintiff's attorney must prepare an answering document for a fantasy trial, a prime example of why lawsuits take so long to prosecute and why the courts are backed up. The defense's delaying tactics discourage attorneys from litigating a sovereign immunity lawsuit.

By the defendant's actions on 11 June, it is evident that this case is nowhere near the end.

The defendant's interrogatories asked for all the doctors Beth had seen in the last five years, and I named 6. Defense counsel then issued each of them a SUBPOENA DUCES TECUM WITHOUT DEPOSITION. YOU ARE now COMMANDED to appear at the defendant's law offices during regular business hours within 15 days of service of this subpoena and to have with you at that time and place the following concerning Elizabeth.

A COMPLETE COPY OF YOUR FILE/CHART, including, but not limited to, office notes, written reports, consultation notes or reports, telephone messages, correspondence, signed informed consent sheets, sign-in sheets, and patient information forms:

All x-rays, FILMS, pictures, scans and diagnostic studies, and corresponding reports of the patient named above are in your possession and control.

Copies of all documents of any kind about MEDICAL BILLS for expenses incurred and payment received on account for services provided for the patient named above, including, but not limited to, itemized statements, office ledger cards, print-outs of spreadsheets, invoices, bills, claim forms, paid receipts, and bank deposit slips.

This subpoena requires you to produce copies of your entire file regardless of whether you consider some documents irrelevant or immaterial. If you do not: (a) appear as specified, (b) furnish the records instead of appearing as provided above: or (c) object to this subpoena, you may be in contempt of court. You are subpoenaed by the attorney whose name appears on this subpoena, and unless excused from this subpoena by the attorney or the court, you shall respond to this subpoena as directed.

How would you, a doctor, like getting a subpoena for medical records on a patient you have not seen for years? It needs to be clarified what the requested information has to do with the lawsuit. However, the attorney requesting these medical records is on retainer to LMHS, and reviewing these records becomes billable hours.

On 30 June, the defendant filed their response to the Plaintiff's Request to Produce—a party requests to produce documents for the opposing party to present certain documents for examination. The plaintiff presented to the Defendant a list of 65 papers.

The defendant furnished requests for policies, procedures, mission statements, etc., without question because they were available to the public. When it came to providing documents of significance having a bearing on the case, their answer was "Object to the question as being overbroad, vague, ambiguous, immaterial, irrelevant and not calculated to lead to the discovery of admissible evidence," was attached to 26 of the 65 documents requested from the defendant.

A request for the production of documents is a litigation stage involving each party collecting and organizing their respective evidence in preparation for the trial. The burden is on the receiving party to provide copies of all requested documents or refuse on privileged grounds.

The receiving party may grant or deny the requesting party the right to inspect the identified records. If the receiving party has that right, why would they furnish documents that may be incriminating? This Request to Produce added 19 pages to the Court record, but only a little usable information.

Some examples of documents requested that the defendant determined to be irrelevant and my answer to why the plaintiff decided them to be relevant.

Requested document:

Written staff education plans were in effect while the plaintiff was in residence. Reason for the request: This document is relevant to determine whether the staff was aware of federal Medicare operating mandates and trained to give medical aid when necessary. Is the nursing staff periodically reviewed to see if they can perform the intravenous insertion procedure and are aware of Medicare directive CMS 20068?

Document requested:

All resident family council minutes or documents recording the council's discussions, plan, or determination during the plaintiff's residency. Reason for request: This document is relevant because these minutes would show whether HPCC informed the plaintiff or her representative of the health risks associated with an embedded catheter.

Document requested:

All reports or written compilations of data about the status or condition of the resident. Reason for request: Condition status reports are relevant because they would have shown if the plaintiff showed signs of severe dehydration that eventually sent her to the hospital in a non-responsive state.

Document requests:

According to Florida Statutes, copies of all reports show staff-to-resident ratios and compliance records with staffing requirements. Reason for request: This is relevant information because knowing the staff-to-resident ratio in May 2017 was low and thus necessitated embedding a catheter to reduce the workload on an understaffed aide population, thus eliminating the need for the aides to help the resident to go to the bathroom.

Once again, what value does a request for documents have when both the defendant and the plaintiff may determine that the records requested are irrelevant?

On 30 June, the defendant answered the 22 interrogatory questions sent by the plaintiff to the defendant on 13 May. The little questions, such as names of officers or other information available to the public, were answered. Still, the essential questions were not—one example of a question and the answer given to 15 of the 22 questions.

Question: Do you claim that any health care provider, including but not limited to physicians who attended to the plaintiff, fell below any accepted standard of care in their treatment of the plaintiff? Answer: Unknown currently, and discovery is ongoing.

Think about this answer. The defendant was served with an NOI in April 2018, and as of June 2020, the defendant is still in the discovery stage to see if any medical provider's care fell below the accepted standard of care. Once again, if the defendant can choose to answer only those questions irrelevant to the plaintiff, going through discovery' is an exercise in futility.

As part of discovery, I was deposed by the defendant's attorney for two hours on Zoom in May.

The deposition was not for information gathering, as the defense's question stated, "Give me the names of some of the people you play golf with." The purpose was to observe firsthand what kind of a witness I would be if the case proceeded to trial. Depositions are costly, paying for a recorder and the transcripts. Did the defense attorney accomplish what he sought by deposing me? Only he knows that.

Let me get off subject here. I started watching a Netflix series on Lenox Hill Hospital in New York. The series covers all aspects of what occurs in a busy hospital. The element that stood out to me was the delicate surgery performed in the operating room and the detailed attention of the doctors and nurses.

Seeing this, Beth immediately came to mind. She loved being an operating room nurse, a position not granted to many nurses because of the skill needed to mesh with the operating surgeon, knowing what surgical instrument he needed next. Beth loved the responsibility and was one of the only nurses in the hospital requested by surgeons to aid in the operating room. The surgeons even let her do the final stitching on significant surgery.

The series also covered childbirth, showing some problematic deliveries, and reminded me of my son's exceedingly difficult delivery. A child she tried to have for eighteen years, suffering three miscarriages and not knowing if the child she had just born would live.

All turned out well, and we had a healthy and brilliant child. She dotted on that child and was his primary parent who read children's books to him from an early age, helped him with his homework, got him through his girl problems, and was the unseen driving force for his being where he is today. He learned baseball and golf from me but knowledge from his mother.

Showing the husbands and wives sitting with a sick or recovering spouse brought back the many days I spent by her bedside in the hospital. Her constant pain, and the feeling of having to pee all the time with no urine to pass, were heartbreaking.

Only a woman reading this can know the pain associated with a urinary tract infection. It is a condition a woman may experience only once or twice in a lifetime, so only a woman can imagine what it must have been like to have twenty-five UTIs in two years.

The series showed the doctor talking to the parents or spouses of the sick patient and updating them on progress. In her last hospital visit, I never had a doctor sit down with me and tell me the end was near. Nurses were the ones who kept me up to date, along with my ability to access and analyze her labs. I reviewed her GFR, which shows her kidney function dropping to stage five kidney failure, and I knew she was dying.

A hospice representative agreed with my diagnosis and determined she was a candidate to be moved to the hospice house, the same hospice she had volunteered for years. She sat with dying patients to allow their caregivers some free time. I now became the sitter. It would have been nice to have a doctor make or agree with my evaluation of her dying, but the results would be the same eventuality regardless of who made the decision.

Chapter 27
Request to Produce

My attorney sent me 270 pages of Defendant's Request to Produce containing 260 pages of insignificant information such as organization charts, mission statements, licenses, and surveys.

There was one significant piece of information, the Census Reports. The Census Daily Detail shows the highest facility occupancy to be 107 residents and the highest Medicare bed occupancy to be 49 residents. On the day Beth was rushed to the hospital, July 29th, the total population at the facility was 96 residents or 90% of maximum capacity, with only 34 Medicare beds occupied by residents, a 69% capacity.

For HPCC to tell me on 2 August that Beth could not return to the facility because there were no beds available was a complete fabrication. HPCC did not want Beth back because she required too much care.

The records also revealed that the facility charged Medicare $9,725 for the 60 days of questionable physical and occupational therapy. I can see why HPCC wanted her out of the facility so they could bring in a paying therapy resident.

The 270 pages provided nothing unknown but increased the hourly rate the opposing counsel could bill the defendant and added another month to the lawsuit. I started an email chain with my attorney.

The latest interrogatories tell us nothing. What is meant by their response to our questions about the standard of care being 'discovery is ongoing'? Does the defendant suspect a healthcare provider may have fallen below the accepted standard of care? You would think the three years the defendant knew of our intention to sue would have been sufficient time to complete discovery.

Discovery has been an exercise in futility since neither party will disclose anything the other party does not know. Since discovery has not shown any issue of material fact, why not move for 'summary judgment' or a 'jury trial'?

He answers: Defense attorneys regularly object to our requests and can make us fight for the records. Before we jump into depositions and fight for records, I would like to involve a nursing home expert to review the pre-suit discovery and our discovery. It will add value to the case but can also offer guidance on how we order and whom we depose.

My response: We have compelling documentation supporting our suit, and I do not believe an expert can strengthen our case. Our most crucial document is CMS 20068. The dehydration issue is a good backup, but there is no way HPCC can dispute the charge that, being a federal Medicare facility bound to operate under the Medicare guidelines detailed in CMS 20068, it knowingly disregarded the mandate described therein. Further discovery should ask only one question.

"Were the facilities management, doctors, and nursing staff familiar with CMS 20068, and did they knowingly disregard the catheter mandates?"

Attorney answer: To be successful or go to a trial in a Nursing Home case, we will need an expert. I am happy to answer your questions to keep you as involved and informed as you wish, but we will not be taking your direction on how to conduct the litigation or the case strategy. A phone conference may be proper to discuss the matter further and use an expert.

In a scheduled 17 June conference call, I will object to retaining a nursing home expert. We have CMS20068, the smoking gun, and records showing the defendant violated that Medicare mandate, contributing to the Plaintiff's death. LGF has had this case for three years, so why are you now calling in an expert?

The defendant's nursing home violated another federal standard in other research. The Omnibus Budget Reconciliation Act (OBRA), also known as the Nursing Home Reform Act of 1987, sets forth national standards of how nursing homes should provide care to residents. One of the improvements in the act is reducing the inappropriate use of indwelling urinary catheters.

Nursing homes must comply with federal requirements to participate in Medicare programs. A nursing home must comply with the OBRA quality of care mandates in caring for a resident to exercise the degree of reasonable care and skill a resident should expect.

Nursing care requirements under OBRA include: Supplying proper respect to those with urinary problems, including only using urinary catheters when appropriate, as outlined in the regulations to prevent adverse consequences of such use. These regulations further support my contention that we already have the 'smoking gun,' the Medicare and the OBRA regulations, and HPCC violated both.

These regulation violations are 'negligence per se,' which refers to an illegal act 'in itself' or inherently unlawful. The action is considered egregious and does not require any added proof of criminal intent. In a civil suit, proving someone guilty of an illegal act 'per se' requires only evidence that HPCC violated a statute and that violation was the cause of the Plaintiff's damages. HPCC has no defense because records show they violated both regulations.

OBRA also states, "Provide each resident with sufficient fluid intake to prevent dehydration." Rushing Plaintiff to the emergency room in a non-responsive state due to dehydration was another charge in our suit. Dehydration risk factors include coma, altered mental status, tachycardia, lethargy, light headiness, reduced skin turgor, and abnormal lab values.

Plaintiff exhibited all of these symptoms. Severe dehydration can cause orthostatic hypertension, leading to shock, and inadequate rehydration, if not accomplished quickly, can lead to painful conditions, including renal failure, heart attack, and stroke. HPCC breached the contract by letting Plaintiff get so dehydrated that she had to be rushed to the hospital. By undertaking a resident's care, HPCC implicitly warrants that they possess the required skill to treat the resident and will exercise ordinary skills and care.

Nursing homes must deliver adequate and proper quality care, which means doing the right thing at the right time and in the right way for the right person. The facility did not immediately react to a medical emergency and did not exercise ordinary skills and care. The general conclusion of all medical opinions is that there is no excuse for dehydration.

The primary purpose of our 17 June call was for him to justify the need to retain a nursing home expert. I told him HPCC's violation of Medicare and OBRA directives on catheters and dehydration should already make our case. That is the case brief for the novice but not for the Court.

Even though HPCC's medical records show they violated both statutes, we cannot make that statement. The statement must come from a medically trained expert. My attorney must prepare the case, assuming it will be going to a jury trial, and thus an expert is needed. I agreed to the $1,500 expenditure.

Chapter 28
Medicare Complaint

Independent of the lawsuit, I needed to find a way to have HPCC sanctioned by Medicare for its misconduct. My solution was to file a formal complaint with Medicare. After many phone calls, I was connected to the organization under contract with Medicare to conduct reviews of all written complaints from beneficiaries about the quality of services not meeting professionally recognized standards of health care.

However, I had one problem: a three-year statute of limitations on filing a Medicare 'Quality of Care Complaint.' Since HPCC performed the unauthorized use of an embedded catheter in May of 2017, it fell outside the three-year statute. However, since I am filing this complaint on 17 July 2020, I can use 29 July 2017, the date my wife went to the hospital in a dehydrated state, as my complaint date. This date now puts me twelve days inside the three-year statute.

On 17 July, I filed three formal Quality of Care Complaints with K, the vendor contracted by Medicare, to investigate such complaints. The first had to do with the dehydration misconduct of the nursing home. The second is catheter embedding, which was implanted for 52 days at the time of transfer from HPCC to the hospital on 29 July. Medicare mandates that an embedded catheter be removed as soon as possible to prevent future urinary tract infections.

Its 52-day retention dose does not comply with Medicare mandates for its removal. The third complaint was what AARP called nursing home eviction or patient dumping. My wife was emergency transferred out of HPCC due to their negligence, a home she had just spent sixty days therein. She was denied re-entry after her hospital stay because the HPCC had no bed.

Their excuse was a fabrication since the Daily Census Report for the day she left the facility showed the home had 15 Medicare beds available. She was denied re-entry, not because of no open bed, but because she was too much trouble to care for and had used up her sixty days of Medicare-reimbursed physical therapy. I claim her not being readmitted was a financial not care decision.

I chose the Medicare complaint alternative because, as is presently being experienced, a lawsuit looking to fault the nursing home for its medical malpractice can take years to fruition. A Medicare complaint is estimated to take up to 60 days, and I hope the Medicare report will support my claim of medical malpractice by HPCC. Following are the formal complaints filed with K.

Charge: Elizabeth, on July 29th, 2017, was rushed by ambulance from HPCC to the hospital emergency room in a non-responsive state. She was severely dehydrated and suffering from a urinary tract infection and pneumonia. The emergency room doctor started aggressive intravenous rehydration, eventually returning her to a responsive state. She was non-responsive for two hours.

Background: In May 2017, Elizabeth was moved to HPCC from the hospital for skilled nursing for a displaced comminuted left fibula fracture. She was also suffering from a urinary tract infection and, for information purposes, had a BUN level of 15. Elizabeth appeared dehydrated in early July, and a skin turgor test confirmed my dehydration diagnosis.

The nursing supervisor was informed of Elizabeth's being dry, agreed with my diagnosis, and told me, "We will get her to drink more."

Showing no hydration improvement, I again informed the nursing staff that her dehydration was worsening, as evidenced by her BUN level being up to 25, with the top of the BUN range being 17. I convinced the nursing staff that she was dehydrated and needed intravenously rehydrated. The nurse said she would administer an IV line and begin intravenous rehydration. Returning the next day and finding no IV line in Elizabeth, I enquired why not.

The nursing supervisor responded, "We tried four times to put in the IV, but her veins kept collapsing, and we discontinued our efforts." The entire nursing staff of HPCC could not perform a procedure learned in Nursing 101.

Their solution to the problem was, "We will get her to drink more." As her condition deteriorated, I told the staff PA that Elizabeth needed emergency room treatment.

She responded, "We will find someone here who can insert an IV line." A week after the first attempt to IV her, the facility did find a male nurse who inserted the IV. However, it was too late.

During this time, Elizabeth exhibited more confusion and memory loss with fatigue and weakness, all symptoms in the elderly of dehydration and possible urinary tract infection. On July 28th, Elizabeth had an appointment with her ortho surgent, where the nurses observed her being so tired that they had difficulty getting her on the x-ray table. She also continues to pass out when left alone in her wheelchair.

The nurses said HPCC should be told that there was something significantly wrong with Elizabeth as soon as Beth returned, and they should examine her. I also informed HPCC that Elizabeth was now weight-bearing for physical therapy. I told the HPCC's nursing staff of the surgeon's nurse's concern about Elizabeth's condition receiving no comment.

On the morning of July 29th, I received a call telling me they found Elizabeth in a non-responsive state and had called the HPCC doctor to see what they should do. You would think the next step would be to get her to the emergency room and not be dependent on the doctor telling HPCC to do so.

Shortly after, a second call informed me that Elizabeth had been rushed to the hospital in a non-responsive state. The hospital found her severely dehydrated and had a urinary tract infection and pneumonia. She was admitted to the hospital for four days.

Claim: HPCC did not adhere to standard operating procedures to prevent resident dehydration, did not respond to the resident's representative that she was dehydrated, and when finally agreeing she was severely dehydrated and needed an IV procedure, did not have a nurse on staff qualified to insert an IV.

Charge: On July 29th, 2017, Elizabeth was rushed to the hospital in a non-responsive dehydrated state from HPCC with an embedded urinary catheter. In defiance of CMS 20068, the catheter should not have still been embedded. Medicare states that a catheter will only be implanted if the resident's clinical condition demonstrates that catheterization is necessary.

A resident receives a catheter and is assessed for removal as soon as possible. The catheter, which HPCC embedded for no medical reason, had been in the resident for 52 days when she was transferred to the hospital. Even though the catheter was inserted before the three-year statute, it was still embedded on July 29th, within the three-year rule, violating Medicare mandates. HPCC should have removed it before her leaving.

Background: I realize a lawsuit has no bearing on this charge, but the language in the suit gives a brief description of HPCC's malicious violation of Medicare guidelines. Elizabeth was admitted to HPCC to treat and rehabilitate displaced comminuted left fibula and left fibula fractures. As part of the treatment for her fractures, the doctor placed a leg brace to immobilize the leg making it impossible for her to go to the bathroom without help.

Due to the perceived potential inconvenience of having to help Elizabeth to the toilet each time she needs to urinate, agents and employees of HPCC inserted a urinary catheter into Elizabeth's urinary tract to drain her urine bladder. To justify using the urinary catheter as necessary, for reasons other than the convenience of the agents and employees, HPCC entered Elizabeth's plan of care, showing she had been diagnosed with obstructive uropathy, a urinary blockage.

Yet there is no mention in Elizabeth's other medical records that such a diagnosis of obstructive uropathy was ever made. This catheter caused Elizabeth chronic pain and discomfort, including the constant urge to urinate despite an inability to do so. Due to using this urinary catheter, not for treatment of any medical condition but simply for the convenience of agents and employees of HPCC, Elizabeth contracted a series of urinary tract infections requiring more hospitalizations due to antibiotic resistance.

Another nursing home finally removed the catheter when they found it served no medical purpose. Medicare CMS 20068 states that if a catheter must be used, ensure the resident receives appropriate treatment and services to prevent urinary tract infections. HPCC violated this mandate, as evidenced by Elizabeth's UTI on July 29th when she transferred to the hospital.

For the next two years, Elizabeth suffered 25 UTIs, 12 of which required hospitalization. Eventually, the UTIs became so severe that they shut down her kidney function, and she died prematurely on July 8th, 2019.

Claim: HPCC violated Medicare guidelines by, on July 29th, 2017, transferring Elizabeth to the hospital with an embedded catheter that should have been removed and communicating inaccurate medical information justifying the catheter still being implanted. One of OBRA's regulations was to reduce the inappropriate use of indwelling urinary catheters. Nursing homes must comply with federal requirements to participate in Medicare programs.

The failure of a nursing home to comply with OBRA quality of care mandates, namely, in this case, the removal of an improperly inserted catheter when transferring a resident from a nursing home, is a failure to exercise the degree of reasonable care and skill a resident should expect from that nursing home. I contend that the July 29th, 2017, failure to remove the catheter falls within the three-year mandate, and said violation should be subject to review by K.

Charge: On July 29th, 2017, Elizabeth was rushed to the emergency room by HPCC after being found in a non-responsive state due to the negligence of HPCC, namely letting the resident fall into a comatose state from dehydration. After a brief hospital stay, I assumed she would return to HPCC, where she had spent the last two months, and they were familiar with her condition and could start weight-bearing physical therapy.

However, the Case Manager told me HPCC could not take her back because they had no bed available. Remember, she had just left HPCC two days ago. I was informed by the Case Manager, off the record, that HPCC did not want her back because she required too much care and had used her sixty days of Medicare-reimbursed physical therapy.

HPCC would rather have a new resident whose sixty days of physical therapy were available. I had two days to find a nursing home bed in another facility.

Background: To summarize the above scenario. Elizabeth was rushed from HPCC to the emergency room in a non-responsive state due to HPCC's negligence. After spending four days in the hospital to recover from HPCC's neglect and having just spent sixty days in HPCC, she was told she could not return because there was no bed available.

HPCC's Census Report of July 29th, 2017, revealed that HPCC had 15 Medicare beds available, thus making the no bed reason false. It becomes more evident that the refusal to take her back was because she was too much trouble to care for and used up all her Medicare-reimbursed physical therapy.

Discharges and evictions lead the list of complaints that state long-term care ombudspersons receive each year. CMS states that once someone becomes a resident, "It should be rare" for the facility to say later that they cannot take them back. An AARP article gives an example of a nursing home resident sent to the hospital for an evaluation, and when the hospital cleared her on the same day, the nursing home refused to take her back.

Their refusal to take her back is an example of what AARP describes: "The problem of patient dumping is one of the most troubling complaints of nursing home residents throughout the country."

"This is a form of abuse by nursing homes that dump these patients to fill their beds with 'better' residents." They further quote the article, which applies to Elizabeth's situation.

"To maximize profit through decreased staffing, unscrupulous nursing facilities try to illegally evict the residents who are the neediest of staff time and require the greatest levels of care." One such method of 'dumping' is for the facility to give away the residents' beds when they are temporarily hospitalized and refuse to readmit them after they are medically cleared to return.

Claim: HHPC should be required to show why Elizabeth was not allowed to return to a Medicare facility after being cleared from the hospital. HPCC should have shown why her non-return was because the facility had no beds available when the Census Report on her day of return showed 15 Medicare beds. HPCC should have shown bed availability and not profit was why she did not return.

A call to the organization I filed informed me that the complaint went into the system on July 22nd, and a review, which will take at least sixty days, has started. I contended that the facts presented to K met the qualifications to file a 'Quality of Care Complaint,' and I believed they would agree with my findings after an investigation by K.

At this time, my attorney gave me the expert's name, an internal medicine doctor who 'will officially author any opinions.' Still unconvinced of needing a nursing home expert, I decided to play lawyer again. I believe this is a 'cause and effect' lawsuit. We know the 'cause,' embedding a catheter in violation of Medicare mandates as documented in Elizabeth's health records, so why do we need a $1500 opinion from a nursing home expert to tell us what we already know?

If an expert is necessary, shouldn't it be a urologist who can detail the 'effect' of embedding a catheter and leaving it in for an extended period? Only a urologist can detail the resulting urinary tract infections, the kidney failure resulting from continued UTIs, and the ultimate result of death due to kidney failure. I do not believe an opinion from an internal medicine physician can make this same diagnosis. My attorney informed me that the case was still a 'nursing home complaint,' not a 'wrongful death suit.' Thus, a nursing home medical expert would prepare a statement; a urologist doesn't need to schedule one.

On 14 August, I emailed him to inquire whether he had received the awaited opinion from the nursing home expert doctor and, if not, to hold up on asking for it. I informed him that I was anticipating a Medicare report that would support our case and be far more superior in value than an opinion from a nursing home expert. I was confident K would recommend Medicare sanctions.

Chapter 29
Case Update

To prosecute this lawsuit, LMHS has retained an outside attorney. With LMHS being a public health care system, they are paying outside counsel tens of thousands of dollars of my money to litigate against me. Therefore, I should know the amount paid to said attorney. On 3 August, I sent a Freedom of Information Act request to their Compliance Department asking for an accounting of all compensation paid to the named outside counsel to date.

On 14 August, I received an answer. LMHS stated that the documents I requested were exempt because they are a part of pending litigation. Locking in on the 'exempt at this time notation, I will resubmit a new FOIA request, asking the same question after the pending litigation.

In March, I had prepared an article for the newspaper but was advised by my attorney to refrain from sending it because it may jeopardize the case. It is evident that not sending it did not move the case either.

The public needs to be educated about the trials and tribulations involved in filing a wrongful death lawsuit against a 'deep pockets' defendant. On 22 September, I sent a 600-word op-ed to the newspaper detailing the Florida Sovereign Immunity Statutes. The op-ed was not published, but I will try again when the suit ends. The op-ed will be printed later in this story.

On 11 September, I received an email from my attorney: "I wanted to update you that I have received the full verbal report from our nursing home expert and expect to receive a written report soon. It was much more than I expected, and he found some things we had not considered. Once I receive the report, I intend to list the expert and use the opinion." which required an email from me.

Me: Haven't we just added a knife to a smoking gun we already have in this fight?

Him: I would say we now have someone qualified under the evidence code to testify that the gun went off and who pulled the trigger. He also found several things we had not considered that HPCC could have or should have done to prevent what happened.

Me: Who sets the order setting the case for trial?

Him: The judge usually has a standard order; he issues it when he sets the case for trial. Either side can ask the case be set for trial after they believe prerequisite discovery has been sufficiently completed for the judge to order a trial. He will review the docket and listen to objections and arguments against setting a trial. The judge can set or deny setting the trial. Usually, the judge will order the case to mediation or non-binding arbitration before trial. We need more to ask the Court for a trial date.

I received the expert's opinion, and it was as I expected, telling us what we already knew. The items he added did nothing to strengthen an already documented case. His report follows: I have reviewed the records provided to me about Elizabeth. The care at the nursing home was: Negligent in keeping the indwelling catheter in despite recurring UTIs. (We already knew this)

The nursing home was negligent in keeping Elizabeth on multiple Central Nervous System acting medications despite her elevated risk of falling. (Not relevant) Infringed on the patient's rights by talking her husband out of transferring her to the ER and not discussing other treatment options with him. (Already known and stated in the complaint) Breached the standard of care regarding incongruency in medication list among providers (Irrelevant).

Did not supervise providers. The patient was seen weekly, with most visits happening before 9 AM, which puts her mental status examination in question. (Not relevant)

I will be billed $1500 for this useless expert opinion.

On 7 October, I received from my attorney an Order Scheduling Case Management Conference via Zoom sent to both attorneys set for 24 November. In the meeting, the attorneys must be prepared to discuss, and here it lists twelve items that are too detailed for me to include here. Also included is an Agreed Case Management Plan and Order that each attorney must complete and agree to dates for such completion.

Chapter 30
Complaint Response

In a 30 September phone call from K, the organization investigating my Medicare complaints, I was informed they had ruled in favor of HPCC. I had three days to request Reconsideration, and I immediately told the clinical reviewer I did want Reconsideration and would furnish my reasons for doing so in writing. On 2 October, I received their written report and will summarize their findings and my response to it in my request for Reconsideration.

Quality Concern No. 1: You were concerned whether your wife was appropriately treated because she had an indwelling catheter and developed a urinary tract infection without a supporting diagnosis.

Analysis and Findings: HPCC placed a Foley catheter to drain urine from her bladder before discharge due to her condition, including her non-weight-bearing status. She had an obstruction, causing urine retention. HPCC tried discontinuing the catheter, but her bladder would not empty all the urine. A urologist was consulted and recommended she keep the Foley catheter in place due to her failed voiding trials and urinary retention.

Based on your wife's record, the peer reviewer indicated it was proper to place a catheter because of her condition, including a urinary tract obstruction diagnosis. It is the professional opinion of our peer reviewer that the services that were the subject of this concern did meet all applicable professionally recognized standards of health care.

My response was that the above finding was incorrect as follows:

Charge 1: Medically unsubstantiated embedding of a catheter. Elizabeth was transferred from GCMC to HPCC on 18 May 2018 with a fractured tibia and fibula. When she moved, records showed she was suffering from a urinary tract infection, and the hospital had removed her catheter. Shortly after arriving at HPCC, she had a catheter embedded. There was no medical justification for such embedding, nor are there medical records showing a bladder scan was performed and found urine retention.

My first question is, why would a catheter be embedded in a resident with a UTI or just getting over one? If thought necessary to embed the catheter, the hospital transfer records would have recommended it.

She complained, "I have to pee, even with the catheter." The catheter was inserted, as per HPCC, because she had a urinal retention problem, but she still had the urge to pee despite the catheter.

After months of suffering from the urge to urinate, I made an appointment with her urologist to see if he could give her medication to eliminate her constant need to urinate.

Upon arriving in the office on July 29th, she said, "I have to pee." The nurse immediately scanned a bladder and found it had been appropriately voided.

The doctor's first question was, "Why is she on a catheter?" I told him I had no idea why HPCC had placed her on a catheter.

His answer was, "I know why; it was for the convenience of the staff not to have to take her to the bathroom or change diapers."

"There is no reason she should be on a catheter, and the longer it remains, she will be subject to frequent and more severe UTIs."

Two pages I thought pertinent to a 24-page visit report are enclosed (Exhibit A). His prediction of future UTIs was right on. When I returned, I informed the floor nurse at HPCC of the urologist's concerns about the catheter and his opinion that they should remove it. HPCC took no action.

She remained on the catheter for the fifty-two (52) days she stayed at HPCC. Even though the catheter was inserted, she still had the constant urge to urinate. Not being a doctor, I think the logical step for HPCC would be to have a bladder scan to determine if she was retaining urine.

She did not have a urinary problem if they found the bladder empty, supporting the urologist's diagnosis. With bladder scanning showing proper bladder voiding, the logical decision would be that the catheter was doing nothing to relieve her urge to pee problem. Leaving it inserted would be detrimental to her future health.

The catheter was still embedded when rushed to the emergency room in a non-responsive condition. In the ER, she was also diagnosed with pneumonia and a UTI. She did not return to HPCC but went to another nursing home (FMCC) with the inserted catheter.

At FMCC, she continued her 'I got to pee' mantra, and a bladder scan found her empty. Having found no justification for the catheter, I had no objection to removing it. Even with the catheter removed, after being inserted for seventy-two (72) days, she continued to experience the need to pee, thus proving the catheter was doing no good.

As her urologist predicted, in the last two years of her life, she suffered twenty-seven (27) suspected UTIs, needing fifteen (15) hospital admittances due to their severity (Exhibit B). One so severe that the hospital could not identify the bacteria growth and sent it to the CDC to determine. She was placed on a PIC line for ten days of antibiotics to cure the CDC-identified sepsis.

Also, in all her hospital admittances, she was placed on an external suction catheter rather than an embedded catheter because the hospital had determined that an implanted catheter was a prime contributing factor for UTIs. With each hospital admittance, her GFR kidney function went from 60.0 in June 2017 to 13.9 in June 2019 (Exhibit C). Eventually, suffering kidney failure and died in July 2019, with the extended embedded catheter being a contributing cause of death.

During her twenty-seven visits to the hospital, they scanned her bladder at least thirty times because of her feeling she had to pee, and thirty times found the bladder to be voiding properly. If HPCC had scanned her in June 2018, the scan would have shown that the bladder was not retaining urine, and catheterization would not be necessary.

I refer to CMS 20068 (Exhibit D), Urinary Catheter or Urinary Tract Infection Critical Element Pathway, which I described as previously shown. HPCC was in direct violation of Medicare mandates on using an embedded catheter. If HPCC had performed the logical, medical function of scanning the bladder to determine if there was a urinary tract problem and found no retained urine, it should have removed the catheter.

HPCC did not follow the mandate of "removal of the catheter as soon as possible unless the resident's clinical condition demonstrates that catheterization is necessary." HPCC was thus guilty of medical misconduct by not following CMS 20068.

Now for her suspected diagnosis. Although there are no medical tests to prove the alleged diagnosis, Elizabeth's 'I have to pee' mantra matches the symptom found in SSD. With SSD, the individual experiences having to pee even though there is no urine in the bladder and no known medical reason for her feeling the urge to pee.

There is no cure, but muscle relaxers, physiotherapy, and exercises may help. Her doctor and the hospital bladder scans show that no medical condition required HPCC to embed a catheter. The following final bit of information comes from a lawsuit complaint:

To validate that the urinary catheter was necessary for reasons other than the convenience of the agents and employees of HPCC, they entered into the Plaintiff's plan of care that claimed she had been diagnosed with obstructive uropathy, i.e., a urinary blockage. Still, no mention in any of Plaintiff's medical records shows an obstructive uropathy diagnosis.

HPCC's independent contract doctors, none being urologists, made the first diagnosis of obstructive uropathy. The test for urinary retention is a cystoscopy or other urinary tract imaging tests (Ultrasound, VCUG, MRI, CAT Scans) to diagnose other conditions that may cause urinary retention. There is no evidence that HPCC gave the standard of care listed.

Also, the Analysis and Finding states, "A Foley catheter was placed to drain urine from her bladder due to her non-weight-bearing status." Non-weight bearing does not meet the CMS 20068 definition of a clinical condition that demonstrates catheterization was necessary. She could use a walker and toilet with the aide's help.

The findings also state, "She was also found to have an obstruction, causing urine retention." Still, none of the tests detailed above were done to identify the site of the obstruction, assuming such an obstruction existed. I have records of her last four visits to her urologist, and none show she had any voiding problems. Her HPCC records show no evidence that any of the above tests were conducted. The diagnosis of uropathy was made strictly on the resident's 'I got to pee' statements.

THERE WAS NO CLINICAL CONDITION DEMONSTRATING THAT CATHETERIZATION WAS NECESSARY AND THUS NO REASON FOR IT TO REMAIN EMBEDDED FOR SEVENTY-TWO DAYS. HPCC WAS

IN DIRECT VIOLATION OF MEDICARE CMS 200068 CONCERNING CATHETER USAGE.

Quality of Concern No.2: You are concerned that your wife was not appropriately evaluated and treated. Specifically, you note her skin turgor was sluggish, and she was dehydrated, a condition not assessed and treated by HPCC, resulting in her being sent to the hospital.

Analysis and Findings: Your wife was on a prolonged stay, which multiple UTIs complicated, and HPCC checked her laboratory values weekly and as needed to check for dehydration. Your wife ate less numerous times, so they gave her intravenous fluids. She received intravenous fluids before her transfer to the hospital because she had slightly elevated kidney function results.

Her electrolytes showed she was mildly volume-depleted but not dehydrated. The peer reviewer indicated dehydration would be evident via a high sodium level. They sent her to the hospital because of a UTI and pneumonia. Based on her records, the peer review indicated HPCC appropriately checked your wife for dehydration, which she did not have via laboratory tests.

The peer reviewer determined that your wife was adequately evaluated and treated. In the professional opinion of our peer reviewer, the services that were the subject of this concern did meet all applicable professionally recognized standards of health care.

Whose records were they looking at because they sure did not match my wife's? When K states that HPCC sent my wife to the hospital because of a UTI and pneumonia, it is readily apparent that it is incorrect. She went to the hospital in a non-responsive condition caused by severe dehydration, and it was the hospital that discovered the UTI and pneumonia. My written response was.

Charge 2: HPCC let the resident become so dehydrated, despite being informed of her condition by her husband that she was sent to the emergency room in a non-responsive state due to severe dehydration. Elizabeth's husband told the nursing staff his wife was severely dehydrated, supported by his performing a turgor test and her increasing CMP BUN readings which peaked at 25 with the high range being 17 (Exhibit E).

When it was evident that increased fluid intake would not correct the condition, it was agreed that she needed an IV and intravenously rehydrated. Returning the next day and finding her not on an IV, I was informed that the nurses tried to place an IV line, but her veins kept collapsing. HPCC decided to do nothing and try rehydrating her by getting her to drink more. If they thought she needed to be IV-infused to rehydrate her, drinking more fluids would not correct her condition.

As her condition deteriorated, I asked that she be sent to the emergency room to be rehydrated and was told that would not be necessary and that they would find someone who could place an IV line. Her condition had deteriorated too far by the time they started an IV, and she was rushed to the emergency room in a non-responsive state shortly after that. She underwent aggressive rehydration in the ER to bring her back to consciousness.

Referring to the Analysis and Findings: States that multiple UTIs complicated her stay. Referring to Charge 1, why would a resident with numerous UTIs remain on an embedded catheter?

As for the statement, "Her laboratory values were monitored weekly and as needed to check for dehydration." I was the one who checked those values and the one who informed the nursing staff that she was dehydrated. To verify this, I refer to her CMP BUN readings (Exhibit E) from 6/26/17 to 7/29/17 ranging from 21H to 25H. The day she was sent to the hospital in a non-responsive state, her BUN reading was 25, with the top of the range being 17.

Immediately after hospital rehydration, the GFR dropped to 8. As for the statement, "She was provided intravenous fluids," HPCC provided her intravenous fluids a few days before being rushed to the emergency room. I documented this false statement when I quoted the nurses "We could not get an IV line in because her veins kept collapsing."

The information, "She was admitted to the hospital for a UTI and pneumonia," were conditions found after admission. She was admitted for severe dehydration and being in a non-responsive state. Aggressive rehydration began immediately upon her admittance to the emergency room.

It is incomprehensible why K did not fault HPCC for not having trained staff capable of inserting an IV line and ignoring the resident's condition until finding her in a non-responsive state. HPCC did not provide standard nursing for the resident as required. By the attached records and discussions with her urologist, I have documented that an embedded catheter was unnecessary, and proper testing would have shown this. The statements for Quality Concern No. 2 are false and must be revisited based on the enclosed records.

I sent my narration and the exhibits to K on 3 October. I got a reply on 5 October. They denied my reconsideration, and I could not believe their reasoning. Following is an expert on their analysis and findings.

Your Quality Concern 1, the use of embedded Foley catheter. A medical record review shows that your wife had a history of recurrent urinary tract infections. Due to urinary retention, she was admitted to the skilled nursing facility with an indwelling catheter. (False) She could not void independently, so she medically needed to keep the indwelling catheter in place.

A Foley catheter reduces the risk/prevention of UTIs regarding urinary retention. (False) In this case, keeping the Foley catheter in place was medically needed and appropriate. In this case, our peer reviewer's professional opinion was that the services that were the subject of this concern did meet all applicable professionally recognized standards of health care.

Quality Concern 2 Dehydration, A review of medical records showed that your wife was closely checked by the nursing staff while at HPCC. Your wife received intermittent intravenous (IV) fluid therapy, and there was no evidence of significant dehydration or renal/kidney impairment during the episode of care. On the day of discharge to an acute care hospital, she had an attack of low blood pressure in the context of worsening mental status.

At that time, her needs required a higher level of care. She was appropriately taken to the hospital. (False) In the professional opinion of the peer reviewer, the services that were the subject of this concern did meet all applicable professionally recognized standards of health care. This is the final decision, and no further appeal rights are available.

I decided I could not let the information in the letter stand without my comment. The first thing I did was find out, despite what was stated in the letter, if another level of appeal was available. I sent the following letter to K in response to their 5 October letter.

You stated this is the final decision, and no further appeal rights are available. Despite this statement, I will find another agency to appeal this decision. In your letter of 28 September, you stated for Reconsideration, "You can give us more information and documents, including medical information, that will help with your request." I submitted four pages of narration and five charts you received on 5 October and responded to them the same day.

You claimed to complete a comprehensive review of the quality-of-care concerns I raised. Your first review took sixty days to complete, and your review of the added information took an estimated couple of hours, as you responded to it the same day you received it. A one-hour review does not meet your 'fully comprehensive review' criteria.

Before I continue, I would like to quote the disclaimer on your referred-to UpToDate website.

"The content on the Up-To-Date website is not intended nor recommended as a substitute for medical advice, diagnosis, or treatment. Always seek the advice of your physician or other qualified health care professionals regarding any medical questions or condition."

Elizabeth followed Up-To-Date's recommendations and consulted her urologist, Exhibit A, who stated, "Asked to see patient for the necessity of indwelling foley." Plan: REMOVE FOLEY CATHETER. She did everything your Up-To-Date website recommended, and the nursing home ignored the urologists' advice.

Again, quoting your Up-To-Date website, "The clinical presentation of a urinary tract obstruction depends on the site of the obstruction, degree of obstruction (partial or complete), and rapidity with which the obstruction develops."

No evidence exists that medical tests were conducted to determine the perceived obstruction's size, degree, or rapidity. Based on his opinion, the doctor at the nursing home decided to embed the catheter with no medical test backing.

Let me do the same since you rely on websites to base your findings. I could refer you to many websites that detail the complications associated with an embedded catheter, but I will quote only one.

From the Centers for Disease Control and Prevention (CDC) website: "The most important risk factor for developing a catheter-associated UTI (CAUTI) is prolonged urinary catheter use. Therefore, catheters should only be used for appropriate indications and removed as soon as possible."

HPCC adhered to neither of these recommendations. They did not, through medical documentation, determine there were 'appropriate indications', and they did not remove the catheter for fifty-two (52) days. FMCC, the nursing home she moved to after being denied readmission by HPCC, removed the catheter.

After being embedded for seventy-two days, the nurse determined that the catheter was doing more harm than good, and he took it out. There were no adverse resident effects, and she was able to void, with much difficulty due to the duration of the catheter, and was able to do so for the rest of her stay in FMCC.

Next, you have a false statement under Analysis and Findings for Concern 1. She was not admitted to the skilled nursing facility with an indwelling catheter. The nursing facility inserted the catheter, a fact HPCC never denied. In the same analysis, you stated, "She medically needed to keep the indwelling catheter in place," but it was never shown, by urology medical exams, any substantiation for that statement. Her urologist recommended the catheter be removed, and the nurse at FMCC did so, and she was able to void and put in diapers.

It is difficult to understand how your reviewer completely disagrees with the medical profession, namely doctors, urologists, hospitals, and your client's CMS 20068 Medicare mandates, strongly recommending that catheters not be used unless medically necessary. If used, they are removed expeditiously. His statement "keeping the Foley catheter in place was medically needed and appropriate" was based on no medical substantiation that supported his 'medically needed and appropriate.'

As for concern No. 2, her dehydration, your whole Analysis and Findings need to be corrected.

You state, "Documentation shows the nursing staff closely monitored your wife." If HPCC so closely monitored her, what accounts for the BUN readings shown on Exhibit E?

What does the first paragraph in the Findings section of your letter have to do with the dehydration issue? I have documented that she did not get IV fluid therapy because her veins kept collapsing, and they could not get a feeding line in. If the records show she got such fluid treatment the few days before her emergency transfer to the hospital, they are false and should be subject to proper agency review.

A false statement states: "On the day of discharge to an acute care hospital, she had an episode of low blood pressure in the context of worsening mental status. At the time, her needs required a higher level of care, and she was appropriately taken to the hospital."

Now let me tell you the true story, which I detailed in my Reconsideration document, which appears the reviewer did not read but relied on a false nursing home rendition of events. On the morning of 29 May 2017, HPCC called to inform me that my wife was found in a non-responsive state, and they were awaiting instructions from the doctor.

HPCC, rather than doing the obvious, did nothing until hearing from the doctor. My next call informed me that HPCC was rushing my wife, by ambulance, to the emergency room in a non-responsive state. The hospital diagnosed her with severe dehydration, and the doctors performed **aggressive rehydration** procedures. She was also diagnosed with a UTI and pneumonia. Does this sound like a resident that was 'closely monitored by the nursing staff'?

The statement, "At the time, when transferred to the hospital, her needs required a higher level of care." She did because she was damn near dead, as for the higher level of care needed. When she was discharged from the hospital, HPCC would not take her back, saying they had no beds when records show that many Medicare beds were available. I found another nursing home on short notice, a facility that did not come anywhere near having the capabilities of HPCC. So much for the 'need for a higher level of care.'

Chapter 31
Newspaper Op-Ed

Despite my attorney's advice not to send the op-ed, I composed in March. My duty was to inform the county's citizens about the Sovereign Immunity Statutes and their effect on them if subjected to medical malpractice. I sent the following op-ed to the paper in October, sticking to the 600-word limitation.

HOW FLORIDA'S SOVEREIGN IMMUNITY STATUTES PROTECT NEGLIGENT HEALTH PROVIDERS.

I am in the third year of a wrongful death lawsuit against a nursing home. In direct violation of Medicare mandates, the home instigated a procedure that eventually resulted in the premature death of my wife of sixty years. However, per Florida Sovereign Immunity Statutes (FSIS), my ability to seek proper restitution is severely limited due to caps placed on maximum damage awards.

Sovereign immunity means that the king, who wrote the laws, can do no wrong, as per old English law. Thus, by falling under sovereign immunity, the defendant can do no wrong and is immune from being sued. However, the parent organization has waived immunity for medical malpractice or wrongful death suits.

By waiving their immunity, one would think the defendant would be subject to significant damage awards if proven negligent at trial. This a mistaken assumption; because the waiver caps the damages that can be awarded in a winning lawsuit to a maximum of $200,000 and makes it challenging to find an attorney to file suit against an FSIS defendant, the waiver also caps the attorney's contingency fee at 25% of the award.

Now let us take a hypothetical case. You go into surgery to have your right kidney removed, but due to negligence on the part of the hospital, the surgent removes your left kidney, and because of their negligence, you incur massive medical fees, or you die. As a result of either or both incidents, the FSIS defendant is liable for a maximum damage cap award of $200,000.

Let me digress and quote a December *Wall Street Journal* article.

This summer, the St. Louis County Police Department paid $750,000 in a wrongful death settlement for a PIT BULL shot years ago during a SWAT raid, even though police claim the dog had acted aggressively.

There is something wrong with this picture when a dog's life is worth $750,000, and the Florida legislature values a human life at $200,000.

Based on the above-described medical misconduct, the victim or their heirs would have no problem finding an attorney to represent them—a false assumption. A medical malpractice suit is very time-consuming and expensive to litigate. Assuming a maximum settlement, your attorney, unlikely due to court-ordered mediation, would collect $50,000 for years of litigation.

FSIS has accomplished what the Florida legislature intended—the act aimed to reduce medical malpractice lawsuits by capping the damage award and attorney contingency fees. Under FSIS, even in the hypothetical kidney removal case, the victim would find it almost impossible to find representation to file suit against an FSIS agency. Many deserving malpractice cases go un-litigated because Statute caps prevent attorneys from taking the cases.

The problem with the low caps is that they deter lawsuits against the covered agencies. It makes the agency less responsible for its actions, less likely to address the litigated medical malpractice, and less accountable to the taxpayers who are footing the bill. Lawsuits are to compensate victims for their loss, correct negligent practices, and reduce the chances that the same negligence will not victimize others. FSIS caps do nothing to ensure these corrections.

After waiting weeks and not seeing it published, I emailed the paper to see whether the article met all the criteria for an op-ed. No answer. I thought it was not published because I used an actual lawsuit reference, so I rewrote the first paragraph, changing it to a generic example and not a personal one. The first sentence now reads.

"If an individual residing in Florida is subject to medical malpractice resulting in major injury or death, and the offender is an agency or agent covered by the subject statute, you may file suit against the offender."

This revision took me as an individual out of the op-ed and substituted an all-inclusive generic plaintiff. I was still waiting for publication. I didn't expect to see it published, so I sent this off to some of my golfing friends.

I submitted the attached 600-word op-ed to the newspaper to educate the county's citizens on the Florida Sovereign Immunity Statutes. In this case, the defendant is the LMHS, a public health care system created by a special act of the Florida legislature. LMHS is classified as an independent special district under the laws of Florida and is thus entitled to the provisions of the Florida Waiver of Sovereign Immunity Act. This act is the subject of my op-ed. I have a law degree, so bear with me when I refer to specific laws and statutes.

The newspaper declined to publish the op-ed, giving no reason. I suspect it is either because it relates to ongoing litigation or because of the sensitivity of the subject matter and the defendant. LMHS does not want the county's citizens to know what the statute would tell them. The present wrongful death lawsuit is in its thirty-second month, with no end.

With COVID-19 sweeping through Florida like wildfire, I, an 87-year-old, am tinder. The goal of the deep-pocket defendant is to see if he can get the lawsuit to outlive the Plaintiff. You may share the attachment with any acquaintances who live or spend winters in the county, informing them they are subject to the statute if treated in the LMHS.

I was determined to publish the op-ed, so I wrote to the top newspaper official and pleaded my case. On 26 October, I sent her the following letter.

An op-ed educating the citizens of the County about Florida's Sovereign Immunity Statutes was sent to the paper weeks ago with no publication. This op-ed is a public service announcement for anyone treated in the LMHS, including doctors, nursing homes, or hospitals.

Not having the op-ed published, I circulated it among many friends with the same response. Like probably 99% of the county, they were unaware of the statutes and could not understand why the paper had chosen not to publish the article to inform the public.

The LMHS would not like the citizens of the county to be made aware of the statute, so the sensitivity of the subject matter may have a bearing on the article not being published. Using the words of my recently received notice of a price increase, "Credible journalism is more critical than ever, and the paper is committed to producing in-depth stories." Failure to publish a public service op-ed does not match the paper's mission statement.

The Florida legislature has accomplished its intended by instituting the Sovereign Immunity Statutes. It has reduced medical malpractice suits, not because the claims were invalid, but because the damage and attorney fee caps make even good cases too timely and expensive for an attorney to take the case. The public should be made aware of this.

On 30 October, I received an email requesting a tagline for the op-ed and a picture. I used the tagline 'Plaintiff in a wrongful death lawsuit' and returned with a photo. The editor told me the op-ed would be published. So, my persistence paid off, and I will now be interested in seeing what response I get from the op-ed publication.

I continued to wait for the op-ed publication, but nothing happened. The op-ed is too controversial or a legal issue. It is an active lawsuit, which may be why the paper declined to publish. It is a shame an exceptionally informative op-ed applies not only to the citizens of this county but also to all the citizens of Florida whose medical system is covered by the statute. They will thus remain ignorant of Florida's Sovereign Immunity Statutes.

Not seeing the op-ed published, I tried another tactic and wrote a letter to the paper's mailbag, where individual opinions are presented in 200 words or less. On 23 November, I sent the following letter with the heading 'Information Suppression':

In September, I submitted an op-ed entitled 'How Florida's Sovereign Immunity Statutes Protect Negligent Health Providers' to the newspaper. The article detailed how the statutes apply to every citizen of the county that use the doctors, nursing home, or hospitals of the LMHS. The law describes the maximum damages a wronged individual can recover from a medical malpractice injury or death and your attorney's top cap of a 25% contingency fee.

Lawsuits are to compensate victims for their loss, correct negligent practices, and reduce the chances that the same negligence will not victimize others. The statute caps need to do something to ensure these corrections. They make the negligent health provider less responsible for their actions, less likely to address the litigated medical malpractice, and less accountable to the taxpayers who are footing the bill. The paper declined to publish my Letter to the Editor because of the issue's sensitivity or the subject health system.

It has been over a month, and neither my op-ed nor my mailbag letter has been published. Two reasons might contribute to their not being published. The first is that the subject matter is too sensitive or controversial since it refers to the local hospital making the newspaper reluctant to publish the documents.

The second reason may be the tagline. The tagline is a few sentences in italics at the end of the op-ed that name the writer, such as a garden topic will carry a tag line 'the writer is the president of the city garden club' and thus be considered an expert on growing tulips. Tag lines are usually people with CEO, president, chairperson, etc. My tag, a concerned citizen or a plaintiff in a wrongful death lawsuit, does not show the writer's ability by title, even though the writer has experienced the statute's effects. My attempts to educate the public on statues have ended for now.

Chapter 32
K's Ruling Appeal

Being rebuffed from appealing K's decision on my quality-of-care complaint, I explored different Medicare websites to search for other options. It was then I found one, Medicare Fraud. The Medicare definition of fraud states, "Fraud means an intentional deception or misrepresentation made by a health care provided with the knowledge the deception could result in some unauthorized benefit to the health care provider."

HPCC's medical description of the events of July 29th, 2017, states, "On the day of discharge to an acute care hospital, she had an episode of low blood pressure in the context of worsening mental status. At that time, her needs required a higher level of care, and she was appropriately taken to the hospital."

The actual events of that day should have read, "Resident was found non-responsive and severely dehydrated and transferred to the hospital emergency room." HPCC's fraudulent submission to K, the quality-of-care investigator, was the basis for their decision that HPCC 'did meet all applicable recognized standards of care.' HPCC's intentional deception or misrepresentation of facts resulted in their actions being determined to be recognized standard of care when a correct representation of incident facts might have gotten them cited for not meeting the 'applicable recognized standards of care.' How do I file a Medicare fraud complaint?

The basis for my complaint is that HPCC committed healthcare fraud by giving fraudulent medical incident reports to a Medicare contractor investigating the quality-of-care complaints against them. HPCC knew when submitting the reports falsely stated the medical events and received a favorable decision by K that the services rendered, based on the false reporting for the incident, did meet recognized standards of health care.

HPCC, a wrongful death lawsuit defendant, allegedly used a scheme to falsify medical reports to get a favorable K report, thus helping their pending case.

My next step was a Medicare investigation of fraud and misconduct related to HPCC's programs. Their false reporting to a quasi-government agency, K, the investigation agency, keeps Medicare from imposing program exclusions and civil monetary penalties because their quality of care not being up to the professionally recognized standard of health care constitutes fraud.

On 15 November, I started calling every Medicare number I could find online. After many, "You called the wrong office; you need to call this office," I finally got to a representative. I discussed how I would go about filing a charge. Most fraud charges with Medicare involve money, and Medicare cannot handle a fraudulent medical statement. K must rely on medical statements made to them by HPCC, and I contend that their words describing the July 29th incident were deceitful.

Medicare's representative stated that a case of this nature was not on his list of identifiable frauds, so he passed me on to a higher authority for review. After hearing my story, they recommended I send my complaint to the Office of the Inspector General.

On 13 December, I filed a Medicare fraud complaint with the OIG using their form.

It states, "Your description of events cannot exceed 1500 words." I sent a description of HPCC's alleged fraudulent actions, a summary of which follows.

HPCC provided misrepresented events summaries to K, the agency contracted by Medicare, to investigate the quality-of-care complaints. Actual hospital medical reports show HPCC's description of events was fraudulent. Medicare guidelines state that K must take the medical reports provided by HP as factual and cannot decide on the quality-of-care description furnished by the complainant. K cannot determine whether the information supplied by HPCC was accurate.

HPCC's description of the events invalidates the authentic medical documents provided by the complaint. Thus K, who is supposed to be an unbiased investigator of fact, is limited to only deciding based on the statements submitted by HPCC. Medicare fraud means an intentional deception or misrepresentation made by a health care provider, knowing that action could result in some unauthorized benefit to the provider.

An example of one event. When found non-responsive, my wife was rushed to a hospital emergency room, diagnosed as severely dehydrated and having a UTI and pneumonia. This information comes from the 83 pages of hospital medical reports covering her five days stay.

HPCC's description of the event furnished to K: "On the day of discharge to an acute hospital, she had an episode of low blood pressure in the context of worsening mental status. At that time, her needs required a higher level of care. She was appropriately taken to the hospital."

HPCC had met the definition of Medicare fraud. Based on HPCC's reporting, K ruled that HPCC provided the recognized standard of health care and thus ruled out the quality-of-care complaint. The benefit derived from the fraudulent reporting was that HPCC did not face program exclusion and civil monetary penalties.

OIG is very secretive and will not acknowledge receipt of a complaint, nor will they tell you whether the complaint meets their criteria for investigation. The only benefit I may have obtained is revealing that a Medicare fraud complaint has been filed against HPCC.

I took my information from the K report and would like to see HPCC's actual submittal of their description of events. I sent my attorney the following email.

Under discovery, can you obtain the quality-of-care complaint response by HPCC sent to K, the investigating agency, in 2020? I have documented two complaints with hospital and medical reports; however, my accounts cannot be used by K because their investigation guidelines are based solely on medical records sent by the provider.

Medicare guidelines state, "They must take the medical records submitted by the provider as factual." A review of some of the records submitted to K by HPCC are not factual. The benefit derived from HPCC's fraudulent statements, rather than an accurate description of the questioned quality of care, could prevent Medicare from potentially imposing program exclusions and civil monetary penalties. I filed an OIG fraud report and will need HPCC's response for backup.

The second bit of information of interest.

AOL News highlighted the following news story a few weeks ago: "TR's cause of death revealed as her partner speaks out." The highlights of the report read as follows. "The *That 70s Show* star died at age 65 from a urinary tract infection. Robert's cause of death was from a urinary tract infection which spread to her kidney, gallbladder, liver, and then bloodstream." Does this incident support our claim that UTIs cause kidney failure and death?

He answered that he could not use discovery to obtain HPCC's response to my quality-of-care complaint sent to K. Florida statutes make such information privileged and thus exempt from public records. I was still not going to be discouraged about trying to obtain HPCC's response, so I tried another approach. Researching K's letter, which denied my claim of inferior quality of care from HPCC, I found what may be a way of obtaining HPCC's response. On 15 January 2022, I sent the following letter to K.

Your quality-of-care review process states that K's decisions are based on medical records sent by the provider, and information sent by the complainant will not be the main factor in your decision. Medicare guidelines state that medical records furnished by the provider must be taken as fact. It must then be assumed that the Analysis and Findings detailed in your letter of 5 October 2020 were derived from the nursing home's medical records furnished by the provider.

Based on the hospital records review of the quality-of-care complaint events, the statements have shown that the words in the Analysis and Findings based on the providers' description of events are an intentional deception or misrepresentation. These actions by the nursing home meet the criteria of committing Medicare fraud. Thus, I must be furnished copies of all medical records sent by HPCC used to make your decision. The requested document does not meet the 42 CFR Part 480 (b) (1–4) definitions of confidentiality since the provider's identity is already known.

A formal Medicare fraud complaint against HPCC has been filed with the Office of the Inspector General at the recommendation of Medicare. Based on the information provided by HPCC, K's final decision is the basis for the complaint. Section 480.103 (b) states that information must be held in confidence and not be disclosed except where 'necessary to assist federal agencies responsible for identifying fraud cases.' The requested record will be significant evidence that, along with medical evidence submitted by me, will aid OIG in any investigation they may choose to conduct.

As expected, I am still waiting for a response to my request. Not letting this issue rest, I decided that if I could not get HPCC's answers to K from K, I would go to HPCC to get their responses. On this basis, I filed a Freedom of Information Request with HPCC, which is covered under sovereign immunity and considered a government unit and thus subject to FOIR. On 26 January, a FOIR was sent to HPCC's risk manager requesting all medical records and nurse's notes sent to K in 2020 in response to the quality-of-care complaint applicable to Elizabeth's care while a resident of HPCC.

Still frustrated by my inability to find an agency I can file a complaint about the investigative procedures used by K as directed by Medicare, I started an internet search. I contacted and talked to many who could not address my concern.

Not giving up, I decided to contact K's home office and emailed the Communications Director, asking him, "Should I file a complaint against K's quality of care investigation procedures with K or with the Health and Human Services (HHS)" the federal agency to whom K reports. He sent me the address of CMS, the agency I should file my complaint. After weeks of hunting, I finally reached the pecking order's top.

Not wasting any time, I immediately sent the following email. Per K's recommendation, I am presenting my concerns questioning the validity of K's evaluation of quality-of-care complaints filed by me with them. The attached details show that Medicare's guidelines state that the medical records submitted by the provider must be taken as fact, and medical documentation provided by the complainant is not a factor in K's decision.

Statements furnished by the provider to K were false according to hospital records of one of the quality-of-care complaints.

My concern is, "How can K be an unbiased investigator of quality-of-care complaints when only the provider's records are used, and records provided by the complainant are disregarded?" The following narration went with the email referring to a K QIO Investigation.

A quality-of-care complaint covering multiple incidents was, along with substantiating hospital records, doctor's statements, and lab reports, submitted to K on 6 August 2020. HPCC nursing home submitted answers to my complaints that contradicted my documented description of events. Let me note one of the quality-of-care complaints. On 29 July, my wife was found non-responsive and rushed to the hospital emergency room by ambulance.

Following are some of the notations taken from her hospital records: The patient is a poor historian and not answering questions at this time as she is tired and unable to be woken up. Unable to perform RO: Mucous membranes are dry. She appears lethargic—poor skin turgor. BU is reading 25. CBC with Diff, Comprehensive Metabolic Panel, and RT ABG is abnormal. She was found very dry in the ER, and the doctor started a borderline hypotensive protocol.

She received antibiotics and aggressive IV fluid therapy. She is currently afebrile—differential Diagnosis: sepsis, bacteremia, UTI, dehydration, intracranial bleed, CVA. CXR shows left lung infiltration and effusion. Mental status improved with hydration. The patient has a urinary tract infection and the left lower lobe infiltrates, consistent with pneumonia. She must be admitted for IV antibiotics, hydration, and further evaluation. My wife spent five days in the hospital, and her medical records for the stay took eighty-four (84) pages to document. When admitted to the hospital, she had an embedded catheter.

Here is the documentation submitted by the nursing home to K covering the same July 29th incident.

"On the day of discharge to an acute hospital, she had an episode of low blood pressure in the contest of worsening mental status. At the time, her needs required a higher level of care. She was appropriately taken to the hospital." Based on HPCC's statement of events, ignoring my submitted documentation, and K's professional opinion of our peer reviewer, the services that were the subject of this concern did meet all applicable professionally recognized standards of health care.

Here is a description of K's basis for making their decision. Our decisions are based on the medical records sent by the provider. The complainant can send information to help us understand your concern, but it will not be the main factor in the decision. Medicare guidelines state that medical records from HPCC must be accepted as fact, and K cannot decide if medical records have information that is not true.

Under K's guidelines, only the statements from the provider, whether factual or not, are to be used. The complainant's quality of care complaints, documented with pages of medical charts, hospital records, and doctor's notes under review guidelines, become meaningless, and the documentation of the complainant is disregarded. Under the above-described evaluation guidelines, how can K be an unbiased evaluator of facts?

There is no correlation between HPCC's description of events and the hospital's documented description of the same circumstances. Medicare fraud is an intentional deception or misrepresentation made by a healthcare provider, knowing that the act could result in some unauthorized benefit to the provider.

In this case, the benefits derived are not subject to Medicare's possibility of imposing program exclusions and possible monetary penalties. Another benefit HPCC derived by getting K to state that the provider, based on the provider's fraudulent statement of fact, did meet the recognized standard of health care. HPCC, the defendant in a wrongful death lawsuit, can use as an exhibit at trial that K determined HPCC met the standard of care.

My wife had an embedded Foley catheter when admitted to the hospital. The catheter was implanted shortly after my wife's 18 May HPCC admittance. She was in an immobilizer brace, which required aide help to go to the bathroom.

It is claimed in the lawsuit that the catheter was embedded not for any medical reason but as a convenience to the aides so they would not have to attend to her bathroom needs. At the time of her admittance to the ER, the catheter had been embedded for 52 days. The following excerpts from the doctor's notes recorded at my wife's ER visit address the UTI and the catheter.

Final Diagnosis: Urinary tract infection without hematuria, site unspecified, dehydration, and lung infiltration were also pertinent to this visit. We will treat sepsis empirically; however, we think this is just severe dehydration. The patient had dementia at baseline but progressively got worse and dehydrated. In the ER, she was febrile but hypotensive, requiring IV fluids. We resolved her hypotension with hydration. UTI appears that it is the colonization of the Foley catheter.

The original urine culture from Foley grew out of enterococcus and yeast. Once the catheter was changed, the urine culture showed normal genital flora. Consult urology and determine why the patient must have an indwelling Foley. Does she need to have a chronic Foley? She went to a new nursing home after discharge from the hospital, which questioned the need for a catheter. After being embedded for 72 days, the catheter was removed, and she was diapered.

Another quality-of-care complaint sent to K was HPCC's total disregard of CMS 20068, Urinary Catheter or Urinary Tract Infection Critical Element Pathway, and I described the directive's requirements. Once again, based on false reporting of the incident in question by HPCC to K, K determined that the services subject to this concern met recognized healthcare standards.

However, her regular urologist, not the house doctor, determined through his examination that there was no medical reason for her having a Foley catheter, and he recommended HPCC remove it. He said my wife would be subject to UTIs for the rest of her life because of the time the catheter was embedded. He was right. Two years after leaving HPCC, she suffered many UTIs, which became more severe, eventually shutting down her kidneys and resulting in her premature death.

Another incident involved HPCC's nursing staff being unable to insert an IV feeding tube to hydrate my wife due to her veins collapsing and thus stopping trying to perform the procedure. This event contributed to my wife being rushed to the ER in a non-responsive state due to severe dehydration. Based on misleading information from HPCC, K stated they met the definition of giving standard health care.

I determined that giving false medical documentation to K, a vendor contracted by Medicare to investigate the quality-of-care complaints, met the definition of Medicare fraud. I submitted a formal Medicare fraud complaint to the Office of the Inspector General on the recommendation of Medicare supervision.

K's value dedication statement reads, "We are driven by a customer (Medicare) first approach and work tirelessly to improve our customer relationships. How can K make an unbiased decision based only on the provider's information with that value statement? Isn't the complainant also a customer?"

"Based on the provider's fraudulent statements, K determined that the provider did meet all applicable professionally recognized standards of health care. My quality-of-care complaints should be reevaluated using the complainant's medical information. Medicare has a copy of the Court order appointing me as my wife's representative, authorizing me to discuss events concerning her."

After sending the letter, I received an email from the site informing me of different places I could contact concerning my complaint. It appeared again that I had struck out in my quest to get someone to address my complaint. I started contracting different agencies as recommended in the email, listened to the 'our menus have changed' for an hour, and punched 1 or 2 to connect to the department I thought might address my complaint.

My usual response was, "We don't handle complaints like this; why don't you try so and so." So and so could not answer my complaint; why not try so and so? The one with authority to investigate my complaint was CMS at HHS, and their email sent me on a wild goose chase to other agencies. At this point, I decided to end my quest to get someone to listen to me. But then I was surprised.

I received an email from The Contracting Officer's Representative, Division of Beneficiary Reviews & Care Management, Quality Improvement & Innovation Group, Centers for Medicare Services—Kansas City. It started with acknowledging receipt of my message sent to CMS QIO concerns. His job is overseeing K and reviewing their handling of complaints and quality of care reviews.

He expressed sympathy for the death of my wife, and I respect your efforts to ensure the care given to your wife was appropriate. Please provide me with K's quality-of-care reviews of your complaint. Now I am at the top of the food chain, Department of Health and Human Services, and if I cannot get some answers here, my quest for redress will end.

On 9 February, I received a letter from CMS and will provide some of the points of interest. He complimented me on exercising my right to request a quality-of-care review and my frustration with K's final determination that HPCC's care met all professionally recognized standards of health care. K has an agreement with Medicare to assess the quality-of-care complaints against providers from Medicare beneficiaries.

When K's independent physician reviewers identify an episode of care not meeting the standards of care, K will help a provider improve upon the area of care that fell short of the expected level so the same episode will not affect future patients. I determine whether K followed the proper processes and procedures in handling your quality-of-care concerns.

My evaluation of K's completed quality of care review is to assess its methods used in responding to your complaint, the inclusion of the information that you filed with your concern and use of the medical records, the use of a proper peer reviewer, timeliness of response, as well as clarity and completeness of response. K's physician review had your concern for their consideration while reviewing the medical records.

CMS has no authority to change a K finding. If you think the information in your records at HPCC needs to be corrected, you can request that the provider amend the record. You mentioned concerns about Medicare fraud and filing a complaint with the Office of the Inspector General was the right path for these matters. I regret that your experience with K did not meet your expectations, but K followed the review process required in my examination.

From what you know of me, I could not let this letter go without a response. I put much work into refuting CMN's last line of the letter. My reply follows.

Let us start with K's letter of 5 October, which describes the following as HPCC's response to my charge that HPCC sent my wife to the hospital in a non-responsive state.

"On the day of discharge to an acute care hospital, she had an episode of low blood pressure in the context of worsening mental status. At the time, her needs required a higher level of care. She was appropriately taken to the hospital." In my 5 February letter to you, I documented, through hospital records, that the above statement was false, and there was no correlation between the above description of events and the actual events occurring on 29 July 2017.

Per your suggestion, I started preparing a Medicare fraud complaint against HPCC to file with HIPAA. I wanted to document my complaint with evidence that HPCC made the above statement. To get said documentation, I requested K send me copies of the response sent by HPCC detailing the 29 July incident, and K declined to send them, claiming confidentiality. My option was to send a Freedom of Information Request to HPCC for the documents sent to K in response to my quality-of-care complaint.

On 13 February, I received two five-pound FedEx boxes from HPCC. The boxes had 1600 pages of my wife's medical records from her stay at HPCC. I spent five hours reading every page to find the statement mentioned above, and the only mention of the incident was the statement "DC-based on census discharge event."

Finding no evidence that HPCC furnished the above information, I have concluded that the report contributed to HPCC was a fabrication of facts by K. If my premise is correct, I was wrong in sending an OIG Medicare fraud complaint against HPCC when K rather than HPCC wrote the statement. It is now up to K to provide documentation substantiating HPCC's information. I realize this is a serious accusation I am making, but the ball is now in your court.

Based on my review of those 1600 pages, I find it difficult, provided K used the same documents, to determine how they reached their conclusions on my other quality-of-care complaints.

Let me give another example of a questionable investigation. On 5/18/17, HPCC embedded a catheter in my wife. On 5/25/17, they found she had a urinary tract infection. I find it incomprehensible that a competent investigator would allow a catheter, recognized by the medical profession as one of the major causes of UTIs, to remain embedded for 65 days.

At the same time, the nursing home tried to cure her UTI, and she still had a UTI when she was rushed to the hospital on 7/29/17. A peer reviewer determined it was proper to place a catheter but never addressed removing it when my wife was diagnosed with a UTI.

The peer reviewer ruled that the nursing home did meet all applicable professionally recognized standards of health care. I may only have a Web MD, but I know that catheters and urinary tract infections are incompatible. I could cite other questionable opinions, but to do so would be an exercise in futility.

On 16 February, at 6:00 PM, I received a call from Tom (not real name), the contracting officer at CMS referred to above. We had a highly informative 20-minute phone conversation. I again expressed my dissatisfaction with K's investigation and filled him in on my pending lawsuit. I told him I appreciated the call and had spent many months contacting various agencies to get to him. Since he is Medicare's representative, there was one topic I needed to give him my opinion on.

By ignoring the faults of HPCC, as described in my letter, Medicare is accepting its actions as acceptable standard medical care. By doing so, Medicare will never know: How many residents of HPCC are on convenience-embedded catheters in direct violation of Medicare's directives on the restrictions of catheter use? How many residents will end up in a non-responsive status due to HP not having a nursing staff to insert an IV feeding tube?

How many residents will be rushed to the hospital in a subject non-responsive state, which HPCC will describe as being sent to the hospital because of high blood pressure? I told him the only action that HPCC would fear more than a wrongful death settlement would be Medicare sanctions and possible monetary fines. These would result in Medicare forcing HPCC to change their health care method and in inspections to ensure HPCC instituted such changes.

Tom stated he did not believe he could provide me with what I was looking for to resolve my dissatisfaction with K's findings. He said he could understand my frustration and desire for my late wife's medical documentation and treatment accuracy. While K performs Medicare quality-of-care reviews, it is not K's role to identify fraud or accuracy of medical records per se.

On 18 February, I got an email from Tom telling me the statement about my wife's transfer to the hospital for 'low blood pressure' was not based on the provider's medical records but was the physician reviewer's assessment of her status before her trip to the hospital.

While I understand you disagree with K's review decision, two independent physician reviewers did a medical record peer review using the medical records and their clinical judgment to arrive at their findings. I realize this may have yet to meet your expectations; however, I am glad you brought your quality concerns to K to review. As mentioned in our conversation, if you want to speak to K's Medical Director about your quality review, I would happily facilitate such a meeting.

To which I responded. I want to talk to the Director, and if you give me his email address, I would like to send him my questions before any conversation. Tom responded by sending him my questions, which he would send to the Medical Director. On 19 February, I sent the following letter to Tom to send to the Director. I am sure it is not what he expected.

At the suggestion of Tom at HHS, I am addressing questions to you concerning the investigation of quality-of-care complaints filed with K. The questions are taken from my review of 1600 pages of information covering my wife's stay at HPCC and 84 pages of hospital medical reports covering my wife's July 29th, 2017, emergency room visit. I must assume K used the same documentation to make their ruling that HPCC met all applicable professionally recognized standards of health care. Let me start with the use of a Foley catheter.

As a contracted Medicare vendor, I am sure K knows about CMS 20068, "Urinary Catheter or Urinary Tract Infection Critical Element Pathway." If not, I would like to quote three elements of Medicare's mandated care plan:

1.   Ensure that a resident who enters the facility without an indwelling catheter is not catheterized unless the resident's clinical condition demonstrates that catheterization was necessary.

2.   Ensure that a resident who enters the facility with an indwelling catheter or subsequently receives one is assessed for catheter removal as soon as possible unless the resident's clinical condition demonstrates that catheterization is necessary.

3.   Ensure a resident receives appropriate treatment and services to prevent urinary tract infections.

Using CMS 20068 as my guide, I would like to submit the following facts and relevant questions.

Fact: Due to the patient's condition, the hospital removed a catheter for urine removal on 5/17 before transferring my wife to HPCC. It is recommended that HPCC do a void study if necessary. On 5/18, HPCC reinserted a Foley catheter with no clinical evidence that the catheter was required, such as a bladder scan.

The first mention of a bladder scan was on 6 June, when it was too straight catheter if PVR was more significant than 300. The Foley catheter was removed and replaced with a straight catheter. No records show the results of bladder scans to justify catheter placement on 18 June.

Question: Being aware of CMS 20068, why did K consider the insertion of a catheter without the resident's demonstrated clinical condition requiring one, to meet all applicable professionally recognized standards of health care? Why didn't K fault HPCC for intentionally violating Medicare mandates concerning using embedded catheters?

Fact: The resident's constant need to urinate despite the Foley was the reason HPCC left the Foley inserted. On 30 May, a bladder scan indicated an empty bladder, but the resident still had the urge to urinate, the first evidence that the Foley was not helping. The Foley was removed on 23 June, but the resident still wanted to urinate. The foley was reinserted on 26 June despite her urologist saying her urination needs continued, even with the catheter inserted.

Even though the bladder was empty, she felt the need to urinate. In other words, she is suffering from SSD and not urine retention. He also made a record notation that he thought the catheter's insertion by HPCC was for convenience and not medically justified.

Question: Knowing the urologist's diagnosis of the urge to urinate being psychological and not urine retention, why did K approve the continued use of the Foley?

Fact: On 5/18/17, HPCC embedded a catheter in my wife. On 5/25/17, they found she had a urinary tract infection. I find it incomprehensible that a competent investigator would allow a catheter, recognized by the medical profession as one of the major causes of UTIs, to remain embedded for 65 days. At the same time, the nursing home tried to cure her UTI, which she still had when she was rushed to the hospital on 7/29/17.

Question: How could a peer reviewer determine it was proper to place a catheter but not address the removal of the catheter once my wife was diagnosed with a UTI and not question why it was left inserted for 65 days? At the same time, HPCC tried to treat a drug-resistant urinary tract infection.

Let's address the dehydration issue. K states that a review of medical records shows that the nursing staff closely monitored your wife throughout this episode of care. Your wife received intermittent intravenous IV fluid therapy, and there was no evidence of significant dehydration or renal/kidney impairment during this episode of care.

Fact: In early August, I informed the nursing supervisor that my wife was very dehydrated and that she should consider IV rehydration. She agreed, and they would start the IV. The following day I returned to find no IV line in my wife. Inquiring why not, the nurse said, "We tried to put in an IV line, but her veins kept collapsing, so we discontinued trying."

On 7/10, I informed the nurse super that my wife's BUN reading was 25 showing dehydration. On 7/11, the Palliative Care Visit notes state. Per husband, when do we feel it is critical to treat pt.'s dehydration, discussed at length with husband? I discussed with the husband should the patient be taken to ER for an IV since the patient has had multiple unsuccessful attempts at IV insertion, thus verifying my above statement.

On 7/12, the nursing notes state, "Level of consciousness lethargic, response slowly to verbal stimuli, obtund very drowsy, responds to tactile stimuli." The doctor's notes from his 7/21 visit state husband is overly concerned about his wife's dehydration. Her mucous membranes were dry, along with dark urine in her foley. Doctor note from 7/2 Dehydrated—will get IV fluids normal saline. The husband requests to return to ER if we cannot get fluids through IV lines.

Question: HPCC was aware of a hydration problem in early August but only inserted an IVF line successfully on 23 August. How could K state that my wife was closely monitored for hydration by the nursing staff?

Fact: On 29 August, the nursing notes state, "Special instruction indication lethargy STAT immediately STAT. Urinalysis STAT immediately indicates lethargy. Monitor Lethargy every shift until the change of condition is resolved. Monitor vital signs every shift until the change of state is resolved. Significant Changes in Condition—Decline in Condition."

At 9:00 AM, I received a call from HPCC informing me they had found my wife non-responsive and were awaiting the doctor's orders. At 10 AM, a follow-up call told me my wife had been rushed to the emergency room, still non-responsive. The doctor's notes for 7/29 read: In the morning, she had hypotension and was given IV fluids. She recovered, but her mentation was sluggish, and she was sent to the hospital at her husband's request.

Is the doctor saying I requested that she be sent to the ER, not his? The Nursing Home Discharge Document—Item J1550 Problem Conditions—Dehydration. K's description of the above events read as follows: On the day of discharge to an acute care hospital, she had an episode of low blood pressure in the context of worsening mental status.

At that time, her needs required a higher level of care, and she was appropriately taken to the hospital. Question: If K's reviewer had access to the same HPCC documents HPCC furnished me, how could they make the above false statement?

Fact: Following are excerpts from the doctor's notes recorded during my wife's July 29th, 2017, emergency room visit. The patient was tired and not answering questions typically. She appears lethargic, has dry mucous membranes, poor skin turgor, and is drowsy but arousable. CBC with Diff, Comprehensive Metabolic Panel, Proteome INR, and RT ABG is abnormal. BUN is reading 25—Diff rental Diagnoses: sepsis, bacteremia, UTI, dehydration, intracranial bleed, CVA. CXR shows the left lung in filtrate and effusion.

In ER, she was found very dry; a borderline hypotensive consistent protocol was started. She received antibiotics and aggressive IV fluid therapy. The patient had dementia at baseline but progressively got worse and was severely dehydrated. In the ER was A-fib but was hypotensive, requiring IV fluids. Her hypotension was resolved with hydration, and her mental status improved. Her BUN at discharge was 11.

K did not do a thorough investigation by not getting the hospital ER reports for the day my wife went to the ER in a non-responsive state. K only used HPCC documents tracking her stay at the nursing home but discontinued the investigation without knowing her condition's effects or diagnosis upon arriving at the ER.

Question: Does the ER summary above sound like the same person K investigators stated was sent to the ER because she had an episode of low blood pressure? HPCC violated Medicare mandates, detailed in CMS20068, on 7/18/17 when they embedded a catheter-based on no medical justification. HPCC should have been cited for this immediately by K.

The above documentation substantiates my contention that K cannot be an unbiased investigator if the said investigation is based on medical records sent by the provider. I documented my original complaints with the doctor, hospital, and lab records, all to no avail. K states that Medicare guidelines say that medical records must be considered facts.

As shown above, those facts should be reviewed for what the nursing home did wrong and what it did right. The reason I am so adamant about the use of the catheter is. Two years after leaving HPCC, my wife suffered 25 UTIs, 12 requiring hospitalization. The UTIs eventually became so severe that they shut down her kidneys, and she died prematurely.

On 22 February, I received a call from K's Medical Director's office asking when I would be available to join a video conference call with the Director, a peer case reviewer, and Tom. I gave them options and set up a virtual meeting for 25 February. K asked if I had any objections to the recorded meeting being used as a training aid for further reviews, and I expressed no disapproval of the recorded session. I then prepared the following preamble for the discussion to tell K why I am so vehemently pursuing this case.

Why am I so adamant about K finding that HPCC did not meet all applicable professionally recognized healthcare standards? HPCC is a Medicare-certified facility that receives millions of dollars of Medicare reimbursement yearly. Any judgment against them would be considered a cost of doing business and a rounding error in their operating statement. Monetary settlements are no incentive for HPCC to stop the practices for which they are being sued.

HPCC can write off any judgment as a cost of business. Still, the facility cannot ignore the one action they fear most: a Medicare sanction and possible monetary penalty. To try to get those sanctions, I turned to K. I presented documentation on two quality of care complaints I felt did not meet professionally recognized standards of health care. My submission consisted of pages of narration and medical records to document my allegations. I then waited months for K's findings of their investigation.

I could not believe K's final opinion, which, in theory, stated that all my quality-of-care complaints were not valid and that HPCC did meet all applicable professionally recognized standards of health care. These standards included HPCC's embedding a Foley catheter, absent medical justification for doing so, and in direct violation of CMS20068 on using a catheter. It included HPCC allowing a resident to become so dehydrated that she was rushed to the hospital in a non-responsive state because the facility did not have a staff nurse who could insert an IV line.

It included a statement initially contributed to HPCC and later found to be authored by K. The information described the resident being transferred to the emergency room because of low blood pressure when the receiving ER notes showed the resident was severely dehydrated and in a non-responsive state. K's statement that the resident was sent to the ER because of low blood pressure meets Medicare's definition of fraud. What I presented as medical malfeasance, K ruled to be recognized standards of health care.

My original submission of quality-of-care concerns was to have K review the documentation. If found through investigation, my allegations were factual, to notify Medicare HPCC did not meet Medicare's recognized standards of health care. K, however, ruled they found no justification for my claims, a weighty decision in my case. I am in wrongful death litigation in which HPCC is the defendant.

If the case should go to trial, K's opinion that HPCC met all applicable professionally recognized standards of care could be introduced as an exhibit by the defendant. The defendant could claim an investigative made by a representative of Medicare found the defendant did meet all professionally recognized standards of care and thus should not be held responsible for the plaintiff's death.

99% of the plaintiffs in a sovereign immunity lawsuit will get tired of the delays and agree to an out-of-court settlement for a sum much below what they would be entitled to get their compensation and move on. However, the defendant was unlucky in this case because I am one of the 1%.

I could not believe K found no validity to my quality-of-care complaints, and I strongly expressed my disbelief in letters. In my latest review of the 1600 HPCC medical records and the 84 pages of hospital records applicable to the 'low blood pressure' transfer to the emergency room, I am even more concerned that I was reading a separate set of documents than those furnished to K by HPCC.

It also became evident that K did not follow up with the hospital records documenting the residents' transfer to the emergency room. My frustration is expressed in these questions.

In summary, K cannot be an unbiased investigator of care concerns if only the provider's medical records, and none from the complainant, are the basis of their decisions. I agree medical records of the provider should be the basis for a decision.

Still, those records must be studied so that their excellent procedures and the wrong procedures documented by the provider should carry equal weight in the decision. K states that their review aims to help providers give better quality health care. They will never reach that goal by praising a provider for providing safe care and not faulting inadequate care.

On 25 February, I had a two-and-a-half-hour video conference with the Medical Director, the Project Director from K, Tom, my representative from HHS, and two nurses. The purpose was to discuss the latest round of questions I had submitted to the Director.

Being K's Medical Director and a doctor, her task was to convince me that K did the case investigation they were contracted to do. She paid little attention to my talking points since most of the discussion was dominated by the Chief Medical Officer of K. I wanted to address the extended stay of a Foley catheter and the dehydration issues to get her side.

She contended that the catheter was necessary because of her urine retention. She talked a lot about her medication and told me her pain medication was known to cause urine retention. The UTI was treated while leaving the catheter in because of urine retention, a more significant cause of infection than the catheter.

Beth's urologist, who stated the catheter was installed for nursing home convenience and not needed, should have removed the catheter. I countered that HPCC had installed the catheter, not him, and it would not be his responsibility to remove it. She counters that she was his patient at the office visit, and he could have removed it. She felt she had justified the extended use of the catheter.

My counter-shot down her explanation. I started by telling her the hospital had removed the catheter before transferring my wife on 5/17 to HPCC with the notation that HPCC should conduct voiding studies. On 5/18, HPCC embedded the catheter, saying the reason was urine retention. However, there is no recording that HPCC performed a bladder scan to substantiate there was urine retention. The Director agreed with me and stated that HPCC was negligent in not showing that HPCC did voiding tests.

I quoted Medicare's directive, "Ensure a resident who enters the facility without an indwelling catheter is not catheterized unless the resident's clinical condition demonstrates catheterization was necessary."

"Ensure a resident who subsequently receives one is used for removal of the catheter as soon as possible unless the resident's clinical condition demonstrates catheterization is necessary." HPCC inserted the catheter, using urine retention as their clinical condition.

No entry in HPCC's records shows that a voiding study was performed to substantiate their contention. Even though the hospital informed HPCC to do voiding studies, the first mention in HPCC's descriptions of a bladder scan is not mentioned until 6/6, 18 days after the catheter was embedded. The Foley catheter remained embedded for the 52 days my wife stayed in the facility, and nowhere in HPCC's records does it show any bladder scan results.

I contend that my wife's constant crying out, "I have to pee," was the basis for the catheter still being embedded, even though her feeling of having to pee was thought to be psychological and not physical. The one bladder scan in the nursing notes indicated an empty bladder, and the resident still had the urge to pee, thus supporting the contention that the desire to pee was psychological. This incident alone should have called for the removal of the catheter.

As for the treatment of her urinary tract infection, the Director stated the catheter was left in because of urine retention, but no documentation shows said retention. No evidence in HPCC records shows bladder scanning studies substantiating their urine retention diagnosis. We ended that subject's discussion with the Director, agreeing that HPCC was negligent in not recording the results of their bladder scans if such scans occurred.

The Director also quoted the emergency room urologist saying that since she had urine retention, to leave the catheter embedded. I countered this by saying there is no documentation that his statement was based on a bladder scan, not just HPCC's medical records transferred with the patient.

Next, we discussed the 7/29 dehydration issue when my wife was rushed to the emergency room. The doctor said they properly hydrated her at HPCC, and a 25 BUN reading was not high, even though the top reading on lab reports was 17. When questioned on the statement by K that the transfer was because of low blood pressure, she said that was one of the causes of her being lethargic.

The doctor spent much time explaining my wife's medications and the exhausting condition they could cause. I could not even get her to admit that my wife was transferred to the emergency room because of dehydration, and she continued to emphasize that a 25 BUN was not a sign of severe dehydration. My counter was why the ER doctor's notes state, "She appears lethargic, mucous membranes are dry, poor skin turgor, drowsy but arousable. She received antibiotics and aggressive IV fluid therapy."

Even though the Director did not consider her severely dehydrated, the ER doctor did. I once again told her about the incident when the nursing staff could not insert an IV feeding line and how the doctor's notes showed the husband was overly concerned about the resident's dehydration. I emphasized that her BUN was 25 when she went into the ER and 11 when she was discharged.

I cannot detail what happened in the two-and-a-half-hour meeting since the Director spent much time describing medications, reviewing medical records, and giving me medical reasons for some of HPCC's actions. K had never had anyone question their actions as I have, and the meeting attendees had no idea that I had enough WebMD knowledge not to accept all of K's claims that the actions by HPCC were within the standard healthcare practice.

I researched long-term embedded catheter use hazards as I told her I would. The consensus is that Foley catheters are strongly discouraged for a prolonged period. Research also stated that one should investigate urine retention to determine if an obstruction is a cause so the doctor could take corrective action to eliminate long-term catheter use.

HPCC never notified me to schedule an appointment with her urologist to examine her to determine whether there was an obstruction causing the urine retention. Every website emphasizes that long-term use of a urethral catheter poses significant health hazards and is a substantial cause of UTIs that involve the urethra, bladder, and kidney damage usually associated with long-term indwelling catheter use.

Catheter insertion would depend on whether the user gets frequent infections and UTIs, which my wife experienced five days after the catheter was embedded. CAUTIs are considered the most complicated UTIs and are the most common complication associated with long-term catheter use. I did my research and stand by my contention that HPCC's use of a long-term catheter violated recognized standards of health care.

It was an excellent discussion, and the doctor justified her belief that HPCC did not violate standard health care. It was her job to explain K's investigation procedures, and she did so. I did get her to admit HPCC was negligent in not showing bladder scan results, provided they did any. My counters to her acceptable actions by HPCC were just as valid, but she has an MD after her name. My first purpose in filing the quality-of-care complaint with K was to have them recognize that the care was negligent and thus fortify my wrongful death case.

I didn't get K to admit that HPCCs' supervision needed to be improved, but I did get enough information that some of their practices may need to be revised. This meeting ended my contact with K. At the session close, one of the nurses came on the line. She said she has never had a husband take so much interest in his wife's health care in her twenty-year career. She said she wanted to compliment me.

K had never had anyone question their findings, nor did they imagine a layperson could go head-to-head with a Medical Director for two and a half hours. The Medical Director's task was to prove that K thoroughly investigated my complaints using medical jargon and hypothetical cases. In her mind, she did; in mine, she never justified K's finding on my complaints.

I thought my attorney might be interested in my conference, so I emailed him. Last week, at their request, I participated in a video conference with the Chief Medical Officer and Project Manager of K, the vendor contracted by Medicare, to investigate 'quality-of-care comments,' along with two very experienced nurses and a representative of HHS. K requested the meeting to answer the three-page letter I sent to HHS, whom K reports, documenting and questioning their response to my complaints.

With this being a first, K asked if I objected to the conference being recorded so it could be used as a training aid for other complaint investigations; I didn't. What followed was something none of the other attendees expected.

For two and a half hours, my WebMD went head-to-head with their MD, K's Chief Medical Officer. I documented HPCC's not meeting what K called "meeting all applicable professionally recognized standards of health care." There is no way I can record all the topics discussed in the meeting, so I will concentrate on the one issue affecting our lawsuit: embedding a Foley catheter.

The MD justified the embedding because of the patient's urine retention. She stated the catheter was left in while treating the patient for a drug-resistant UTI because urine retention was a greater infection risk than the catheter. The MD agreed that a bladder scan was the standard medical procedure for documenting urine retention. HPCC nurses' records show they took only one scan long after the catheter was embedded.

That scan stated, "bladder scan indicates empty bladder." Based on the patient's urge to pee, the catheter remained embedded. HPCC paid no attention to the patient's urologist's statement; it was his opinion that the catheter was implanted for convenience, the patient's urge to pee was psychological and not physical, and the catheter should be removed. On 6 June, the first order was issued for a bladder scan every six hours, but no records show the results of those scans.

The order ended on 12 June, and there are no other orders to bladder scan after that. I informed the MD that the hospital had removed the patient's catheter on 17 May before transferring her to HPCC, suggesting that the nursing home conduct bladder scans. On 18 May, HPCC embedded the catheter, violating Medicare CMS 20068 guidelines. By HPCC not doing a bladder scan on 18 May, they did not document a clinical condition needing the embedding of a catheter.

Not doing bladder scans during the duration of the embedded catheter did not show that catheterization was necessary. After my dissertation, the MD agreed HPCC was negligent in not recording the results of bladder scans, provided they had taken them. The MD grudgingly agreed there was no documented clinical reason for the catheter to remain embedded for the 52 days the patient was at HPCC.

Quoting 'Medscape,' Using a Foley catheter for a prolonged period is strongly discouraged because these catheters pose significant health hazards.

Catheters are a substantial cause of UTIs, and untreated symptomatic UTIs may lead to urosepsis and death.

I was hoping my submitting my complaint to K would get K to issue Medicare sanctions and possible monetary penalties against HPCC for apparent violations of Medicare mandates. The one action HPCC would fear more than a judgment. Such sanctions would generate publicity and subject them to increased Medicare inspections to ensure they corrected the actions litigated. I was hopeful K would request such sanctions from Medicare, but my quest was not to be.

After two and a half hours of disagreeing with the Chief Medical Officer's defense of HPCC, going to trial would be easy. By ignoring the faults of HPCC, as I described, Medicare accepts their actions as acceptable standard medical care. By doing so, Medicare will never know how many residents of HPCC are on convenience-embedded catheters in direct violation of Medicare's directives on the restrictions of catheter use.

Chapter 33
Reminiscence

One of my clients talked about selling his declining health father's car, which reminded me of the most painful task I had to perform. Beth was always an independent woman. When we bought our first home in Florida in 2002, she decided we could not be a one-car family and needed her wheels. So, we went car shopping on a trip back to New York. The trip took little time. She saw the car in the showroom she wanted at the first dealership we walked into. It was a silver Pontiac TransAm with a sunroof.

We made the deal, and she had her wheels. That fall, she drove it back to Florida, following me. A scary incident happened on the trip when an eighteen-wheeler ran me off the road into the shoulder resulting in dirt and dust flying while I recovered with no damage. We had to get off at the following interchange so she could calm down. We had no radio or cell phone, so she could not contact me after the incident.

Now that we were residents of Florida, she was happy to get her car and the independence that went with it. She could share our one car there since she only spent four months a year in Buffalo. We arranged that she would fly to Buffalo in June and back in October while I drove both ways.

In 2017 after her fall and failing health, it was evident she would never drive again. I decided to sell her twenty-year-old car, which looked as good as when it came off the showroom floor and had only 16,000 miles. I showed it to one of my golfer friends, and he bought it immediately. When sold, it broke Beth's heart. If the car was in the garage, even though she knew she would never drive it again, it was there.

Her independence was still just outside the door. When the garage was empty, she realized her freedom went with it. She would now have to depend on others to do the tasks she enjoyed doing herself. Her hours of shopping trips by herself, eating lunch out, and usually buying something for me I did not need.

They were gone. Like I am sure many others have felt, her life as she knew it was over for her. I can never forget her silent weeping as the car exited the garage and drove down the street. Her life had ended, and she would not forgive me for selling her car.

Chapter 34
Case Management Plan

Here is a sample of one of the documents submitted to the court necessary to move a lawsuit to trial. It explains why a journey through the halls of justice is not a straight line but follows a twisting road.

In October 2020, the court issued an 'Agreed Case Management Plan, and Order' listing dates the plaintiff and defendant must submit agreed-upon events to the court. Following is an example of the first event with dates and responses with the schedule of events listing going to October 2021. The first event is the Disclosure of Fact Witnesses.

My attorney listed eight people by name, and any witnesses identified in depositions and discovery responses and expanded upon that list with the following:

Plaintiff reserves the right to call all witnesses, including expert witnesses, listed by any party to this lawsuit, including, but not limited to, those identified in Defendant's Expert Witness List.

Plaintiff reserves the right to call impeachment and rebuttal witnesses deposed in this case.

Plaintiff reserves the right to object to any witnesses listed by Defendant and amend this Witness list should witnesses be identified through discovery after the service date herein or at trial.

Plaintiff reserves the right to call to testify at trial those treating physicians and other health care providers upon whom they rely after the service date on this Witness List for treatment.

All treating physicians, nurses, rehabilitation therapists, occupational therapists, and other persons engaged in providing Plaintiff medical care.

Plaintiff reserves the right to add more witnesses to this Exhibit List before trial.

All witnesses listed on Defendant's witness list.

All persons listed on any other party's Witness and Exhibit Lists, whether still a party at trial.

All supervisors and custodians' records of Defendant's employer.

My counsel must list everyone he could call because the defense could object to their being called if he contacts a witness not listed above.

In addition to the Witness list, there is an Exhibit List.

All records of the healthcare providers listed above.

All applicable Florida Statutes and County Ordinances.

Those exhibits are necessary for impeachment purposes.

All exhibits listed on any other party's Witness and Exhibit Lists.

Medical records of Plaintiff.

Hospital records of Plaintiff.

X-rays, MRI films, CT scans, and other Plaintiff diagnostic tests.

Collateral source policies and records about Plaintiff.

Income tax returns and insurance records about Plaintiff.

Clinical Practice Guidelines and Associated Publication of the US Public Health Service about Plaintiff's condition.

All depositions that were taken in this matter.

Any Answers to Interrogatories.

Any Responses to Requests for Production.

Any records identified by Defendant.

Any pleadings contained in the court file.

Any documents created by Defendants, including those kept as part of Plaintiff's normal business activities and medical records.

All exhibits listed on Defendant's Exhibit List.

Any all-anatomic charts, diagrams, drawings, and models created by Defendant for Plaintiff.

All photographs and literature used by Defendant's Experts and Defendant.

Burial records of Plaintiff.

Records of the US Social Security Administration.

Plaintiff reserves the right to supplement this Exhibit List later.

The defendant must also file a 'Plaintiff's Witness and Exhibit List.'

One last example of a document request. On 25 February, Plaintiff issued a 'Plaintiff's Northup Request to Produce' "requesting that Defendant, within 30 days, furnish copies of all affidavits and transcripts of testimony given by any of the experts identified by Defendant whom Defendant intends and have indicated they intend to call as witnesses on Defendants behalf at the trial of this action and other documents intended solely for witness impeachment, which are in possession of the Defendant and which the defendant reasonable expect or intend to use at the trial of this action to impeach the Plaintiff's respective experts." This is the actual lengthy sentence from the document.

I could continue to describe the document following document. Still, I have given a picture of the documentation necessary to prosecute a lawsuit, especially one that will never see the inside of a courtroom. The defense attorney intends to use the preparation of trial documents to slow-walk this case to what we know will be settled in court-ordered mediation. By the defense doing so, he runs up his retainer fee and, simultaneously, the expenses of the Plaintiff's attorney to prepare the same documents at a fixed contingency fee.

As of this date, eighty-two documents have been submitted to the court, and they are still determining what additional documents are to come.

From now until August's mediation, the only activity will be the attorneys' exchanging requests for documents through the court. Due to COVID-19, mediation scheduled for June has been moved to 3 August.

On 10 May, my attorney informed me he would like to add a urologist to his list of experts, which I suggested when he hired the $1,500 geriatrics specialist. A urology specialist will be a costly undertaking.

On 19 February, my probate attorney submitted a new document informing the court that the petitioner cannot file a Final Accounting and Petition for Discharge within the time frame specified in Florida Probate Rule 5.400 because a wrongful death lawsuit is being pursued.

The petitioner estimates that it will be possible to file a Final Accounting and a Petition for Discharge on or before 1 March 2022. It appears my probate attorney sees no end to the suit anytime soon.

Chapter 35
Medicare Recovery Right

On 16 April 2021, I received a letter from Medicare's Benefits Coordination and Recovery Center (BCRC) informing me of Medicare's priority right of recovery as defined under the Medicare Secondary Payer provision. It states that Conditional Medicare payments that we believe are related to your case for the Date of the Incident listed above have been made. (18 May 2017) These conditional payments are subject to reimbursement to Medicare from proceeds you may receive under a settlement judgment, award, or other compensation.

To date, and based on the available information, Medicare has identified $55,562.43 in conditional payments that we believe are associated with your case. Enclosed is a listing of claims that make up this total.

Please review this listing carefully and let us know if this list needs to be updated as soon as possible. (For reader information, on the 26 pages, there were 200 incidents listed with 715 DX codes, the codes used to identify a procedure so that Medicare could pay the doctor for his service. I can determine whether the charge applies to Medicare's conditional payments by defining each DX code. More on this later.)

Attached was a Payment Summary comprising 26 pages of medical charges BCRC considered applicable to our case. The listing covers medical billings from 5/18/2017 through 4/19/2019.

"If you believe the enclosed itemization of conditional payments is incomplete, inaccurate, or that you are not responsible for repaying Medicare for these payments, please provide written documentation along with an explanation to support your dispute/rebuttal."

This letter says that I would be responsible for paying Medicare $55,562.34 taken from any settlement I receive from the lawsuit. Please note that the conditional payments Medicare wanted from me were not paid to me but to the hospital. My interpretation is that the hospital gets to keep its conditional costs, but I must repay Medicare the conditional payments they paid the hospital. Is there something wrong with this picture? To comply with BCRC's request and make the payments, my only redress would be to sue the hospital to recover the conditional costs.

On 19 April, I called BCRC for answers to several questions about the information in their letter. After going through punches one and two, I finally got to a Recovery Department representative. After giving her all the identification required, she asked what she could do for me. I informed her I had questions concerning some of the statements in the letter.

She told me she could not give me the information, even though the letter was addressed to me, because I was not authorized for her to disclose the case information. The only way I could get the info was to fax them a death certificate showing I was the beneficiary's spouse. So, for the third time, I faxed a copy to BCRC.

Later, after giving them time to get the death certificate, I called again. Rather than detail my experience, I will show you a copy of the letter I sent to BCRC on 23 April, showing the conclusion of my investigation.

To comply with your request, "I will review the listing carefully and let you know as soon as possible if the listing is incorrect." To help me submit an expedited review, I need clarification on subjects in the letter from BCRC.

Relying on your, "If you have any questions concerning this matter, please contact the Benefits Coordination & Recovery Center." In a call to BCRC on 19 April, I was told they could give me no information until the center received a copy of the death certificate. I faxed a certificate on 19 April. A return call to BCRC informed me that it took 48 hours for the fax to reach the center.

In a call made 48 hours after I faxed the certificate, I was told it would take up to 45 days to vet it, and they could only give no information after completing the vetting process. A request to speak to a supervisor resulted in the representative hanging up on me. So, I decided to respond to their letter without BCRC's help.

It is evident to me, based on the medical charges you state, "We believe are related to your case," that BCRC has an incorrect interpretation of 'Date of Incident.' I can correct your report by getting a description of your incident date, an item I was trying to get in my abruptly ended information request. I will give the correct version of the incident without having your understanding of the incident.

The resident entered HP Care Center (HPCC) from the hospital with a displaced comminuted fracture of the left fibula and fibula. HPCC placed the leg in a brace to immobilize the leg, thus preventing her from urinating without help. Due to the potential inconvenience of having to help the resident to the bathroom each time she urinated, HPCC violated Medicare guidelines on the restricted use of an embedded catheter and, on 18 May 2017, implanted a catheter.

Again, in violation of Medicare guidelines, the catheter remained embedded for 72 days. After discharge, due to the use of the catheter by HPCC for no known medical reason, the resident developed more urinary tract infections which eventually became antibiotic-resistant. The many UTIs progressively reduce her kidney function resulting in total kidney shutdown and her eventual death. Although the incident started on 18 May 2017, the medical ramifications did not become evident until many months later, when those ramifications incurred medical costs.

The Notice of Intent was not filed with the courts, naming HPCC as Defendant, until 13 April 2018. All conditional payments made before that date should not be included and thus not fall in Medicare Secondary Payer provisions. The new Date of the Incident should be 13 April 2018 to show claims that Medicare has paid conditionally. A review of the Payment Summary shows that $43,382 of those charges were for the rehab facility, rehab doctors, physical therapy, and pain management to treat the fractured tibia and should not be charged to the corrected incident report.

In reviewing the Payment Summary, I have identified only $9,966 charges that may apply to the correct incident. I need to know the DX codes accompanying these charges to verify that they are for treating urinary tract infections. Requesting a copy of the DX codes was one of the questions I still need to ask. Therefore, the Payment Summary of conditional payments shows $45,596 of costs that I am not responsible for repaying Medicare.

An explanation to support my dispute will require BCRC to send me the medical documentation used by you to support the charges shown on the Payment Summary. I will also need a listing of all the DX codes on the Payment Summary to help me review the documents furnished. Since the beneficiary passed away in August 2019, I question why Medicare is "still investigating this case file to obtain any other outstanding Medicare conditional payments."

With a lawsuit scheduled to resume in June, BCRC must furnish me with a final accounting by the end of May. I will consider the $9,966 as BCRC's acceptable final accounting if such accounting is not received.

Seeing that my attorney was not copied on the Medicare information, I e-mailed him to inquire whether he had filed a Proof of Representation with BCRC. In a return e-mail, he sent me a letter showing they had sent it to Medicare on 5 September 2017.

Seeing the letter, I knew where BCRC produced the $55,000 conditional payment figure. The letter states, "Please be advised this firm represents Beth for injuries sustained in a Florida accident on 18 May 2017." The letter used the fractured tibia as the accident, but, as I stated in the letter sent to BCRC, the broken leg was not the incident being litigated.

I told my present counsel that I had notified my second counsel on 4/4/17 that Medicare was working with an incorrect incident date, namely a broken leg. Medicare requested that the incident date be corrected so they do not continue to summarize charges irrelevant to the case. Not surprisingly, council number two did not inform Medicare of the updated incident description, so they continued collecting $55,000 of condition payments from the 5/18/17 broken leg incident.

The letter mentioned above states, "Accordingly, this letter is to request under Florida Statute 768.76(6), that Medicare conduct a review of their records to determine if benefits paid on Beth's behalf were a result of the injuries she sustained on the date as mentioned above."

By statute, Medicare must provide this information within thirty days of receipt of this certified mail correspondence, specifically, "The provider of collateral sources will waive any right to subrogation or reimbursement unless it provides the claimant or claimant's attorney a statement asserting payment of benefits are right of subrogation or reimbursement within 30-days following receipt of the claimant's notification to the collateral sources provided." This is a typical autocratic explanation of why Medicare is sending me all the charges to date.

I noticed my counsel was not copied on the information coming from Medicare, so I e-mailed him the following. Not being copied on BCRC's 4/14/21 letter means you are not recognized as my attorney, who may receive information from BCRC. If the 9/5/17 letter is the only notification given to Medicare, it has expired. The Consent Form is only suitable for a limited amount of time.

Medicare will not release information from a beneficiary's records without proper authorization. You need to issue a new Consent Form to be able to discuss matters with BCRC, along with a Proof of Representation Document. You need to change the accident date and description in any recent filing. His answer is to let us see the result of your letter to BCRC before we continue.

On 6 May, I got a response from Medicare to my letter. They agreed with some of my logic and reduced the condition payments from $55,562 to $23,135. However, I disagreed with the medical expenses on their revised listing, so I again decided to file my objections to the listed occurrences. On 14 May, I finally accessed BCRC by phone and spent 41 minutes discussing their Beneficiary Conditional Payment Letter.

The result of the discussion was that for me to dispute conditional payments, I would have to address every one of the 715 charges shown on the Payment Summary and explain why the charges shown are not considered part of the lawsuit and should not be applicable. Based on these instructions, I did my investigation and, on 11 May, sent BCRC a summary of my findings. I will give some of the highlights.

The first task was to inform BCRC that they used the wrong incident date, 18 May 2017, and description. I told them that was the date Elizabeth was transferred from the hospital to HPCC with a fractured tibia and fibula for rehabilitation. The fractures resulted from a fall at home and are not the basis for the lawsuit. It was the day the litigated catheter insertion occurred, but the effects of that procedure, and the condition payments, would not become evident for many months.

I informed them that the subject of the litigation is a Wrongful Death Suit due to kidney failure. The incident date should be 11 June 2019, when hospital doctors diagnosed kidney failure and treatment began. I use this data following Medicare guidelines which state, "When an incident is not evident over some time, the date of the incident is the date the incident became evident."

I then started my investigation of the $55,562.34 of conditional payments that BCRC 'believe are associated with your case.' Every one of the payment charges shows the provider's name, the DX code, the dates, and the payment amount. To do a thorough evaluation, I would have to know the DX code description, and when I requested such a listing from BCRC, I was informed to look them up myself.

A DX code is the number the doctor or hospital uses to identify what condition the patient is being treated for and is the number submitted to Medicare for payment. I went online and found a website entitled Code Comprehensive Search. By typing in the DX code, I would get a definition of the diagnosis the code represented.

For instance, I482 was the code for atrial fabulation, which would then be the primary code. In some cases, like hospital visits, the primary code could be followed by many subcodes. An example, one of the charges had twenty-one subcodes. Rather than investigating every sub-code, I informed BCR that my investigation was based on the primary code used.

Based on the primary DX code, the body of my letter explained whether the charge applied to the case or not. Rather than describing my findings, I will just cut to the chase and give you my ending letter conclusion. In my investigation of the 200 primary DX codes listed as condition payments detailed on the Payment Summary Sheet, I find NONE of the $55,562.34 BCRC referred to as conditional charges apply to the incident.

On 3 May, I got a response from BCRC stating they accepted my revised date of the incident being 11 June 2019 and had removed $55,562.34 from the associated conditional payments. They now issued me a new Payment Summary with two pages of charges of conditional payments corresponding with the revised date of the incident totaling $6,578.89.

I am sure BCRC has never had anyone question their conditional payments summary as I have. Still, my efforts have resulted in a $48,984 reduction in conditional costs I would be required to reimburse Medicare. Being on a roll, I decided to push my luck further and, on 3 June, sent BCRC the following letter.

Plaintiff—Elizabeth, Defendant—LMHS. The DX code N179, kidney failure, verifies my contention that 11 June should be the incident date. I would now like to educate you on Florida's Sovereign Immunity Statutes. BCRC has submitted to Plaintiff a Beneficiary Conditional Payment Letter saying Medicare has priority right of recovery of conditional payments for Medicare Part A paid to Defendant, but recoverable from Plaintiff. In a typical lawsuit, Plaintiff would include these conditional payments in the final settlement.

Those monies would then be sent to BCRC by Plaintiff to meet their obligation. However, this is not a typical lawsuit.

This lawsuit falls under Florida's Sovereign Immunity Statutes, and Defendant is considered a sovereign immunity entity. Defendant has a maximum liability of $200,000 to cover the pain and suffering portion of a settlement. Under the Statute, Defendant is immune from any other claims, such as conditional Medicare payments, against them. To pay the priority right of recovery claimed by BCRC, Plaintiff would have to take that amount from its pain and suffering settlement.

In summary, Plaintiff must pay Medicare the conditional payments made to Defendant, who gets to retain the conditional payments made to them. BCRC may be protecting Medicare's interest but, in this case, ignoring the claim of the Plaintiff who pays into the Medicare system. Under the above scenario, Defendant wins, Medicare wins, and Plaintiff, whose wife died because of Defendant's wrongdoing, is the big loser.

The logical recovery of Medicare conditional payments in a Florida Sovereign Immunity Statutes case would be for BCRC to direct bill the Defendant for the costs they received that fall under Medicare's priority right of recovery. Plaintiff's attempt to recover those payments from Defendant would be denied because of the Sovereign Immunity Statutes. Plaintiff thus files for a recovery waiver.

On 17 May, I received a letter from an organization called O, a part of United Health. They were to pursue a recovery of the medical benefits paid arising out of the captioned injury. In other words, they, like Medicare, seek to recover the 20% of medical benefits AARP has paid on behalf of your dependent for treatment of injuries sustained. The letter attached is a two-page, 82-occurrence description of every payment made by AARP from May 2017 through April 2019, with costs ranging from $2.36 to $4,606.00. It was then my task to review the 82 charges and highlight those I disagreed with. The total charges O was seeking to recover totaled $9,644.69. The following letter was my reply.

Let me start with your incorrect Date of Injury. The subject of the present litigation is a wrongful death lawsuit brought on by kidney failure. Medicare states that where an incident is not evident over a period, the incident date is the date the incident became evident. Thus, the incident date is 11 June 2019, when doctors diagnosed kidney failure, and treatment started.

All medical payments shown on the Summary for AARP do not apply to the case. Medicare's BCRC, agreeing with the new 11 June 2019 incident date, should remove all conditional payments from the Beneficiary Condition Payment Letter before that date. I request a corrected copy of the subject letter showing the removal of all stated charges.

On 18 June, I received a BCRC letter telling me I could not file a request for a Medicare waiver of conditional payments. A waiver cannot be considered until I receive a formal letter requesting recovery of Medicare's payment. Medicare will not issue a formal letter until informed of a case settlement.

At the same time, I received another copy of a Payment Summary Form that shows BCRC has designated $6,578.89 as the total condition payment I owe to Medicare based on the 11 June date. I was hoping my request for a waiver would keep me from analyzing the payment summary, but I now have to review all the charges again and show those I don't consider applicable. I identified every DX code shown on the overview and submitted the following letter to BCRC on 22 June.

Subj: Dispute of Conditional Payments Shown on 6/16 Payment Summary Form. My request for a waiver of payment would keep me from having to analyze your enclosed Payment Summary Form. Until a formal letter requesting recovery has been received, I must correct your identified conditional payments. The following summary documents that your $6,578.89 total reimbursement amount is incorrect, which BCRC believes is associated with my case, and I dispute it as documented below.

The litigation is a wrongful death lawsuit based on kidney failure believed to be caused by the medical malfeasance of a nursing home. Thus, the conditional payments made by Medicare should be for hospital and doctor's billing to treat said kidney failure. According to ICD10Data.com, codes N17 through N19 are billable/specific ICD-10-CM codes that can indicate a diagnosis of renal failure for reimbursement purposes.

N18.9 specifies Chronic Kidney Disease, Unspecified, and N19 identifies Unspecified Kidney Failure. TOS 60 for GCMC shows 20 different DX codes, of which only two carry the codes N179 and N184 and a code I129 that may be applicable. I will give you an example of some of the other 17 codes listed. F0281 Dementia, F411 Generalized anxiety disorder, R630 Anorexia, Z932 Ileostomy status, and Z66 DNR. Conditional payments made to these codes do not apply to the date of the incident issue.

Not knowing the dollar value assigned by the hospital for each code, I can only assign code values by dividing the $5,833.96 by the 20 codes giving me a code value of $291.70 for each DX code. Since I found only three codes associated with renal failure, the $5,833.96 hospital conditional payment for the incident should be reduced to $875.10.

Now for the individual doctor's conditional payments. For EG, he lists four DX codes with only N179, kidney failure being applicable. The other codes, I10 Hypertension, I4891 A-fib, and N390 UTI non-specified, are inappropriate. His billing goes from $177.71 to $44.43. For Dr. RK, only one of his two codes, N179, is applicable, reducing his billing from $24.27 to $12.14.

For example, the other code used is unspecified N390 degenerative nervous system disease. The other doctors have identified their codes as N179 and N184, which are associated with acute kidney failure, and their billing of $542.87 could fit the criteria of conditional payments. The above corrections reduce the $6,578.89 condition payments shown on the 16 June 2021 Payment Summary Form to $1,474.54. I am available to discuss my billing logic upon request.

After sending the above letters disputing BCRC's conditional payments, I finally accomplished what I intended to do.

On 12 July, I got a letter from BCRC stating: "After reviewing the claims in question, we agree with the dispute, and the case has been adjusted accordingly." In other words, the case has been closed, and the original $55,562 conditional payments, once owed to Medicare by me, have been reduced to zero.

It is unprecedented that BCRC would waive conditional charges before a case settlement and issue a formal letter requesting recovery of Medicare's costs. I am convinced that my knowledge of the DX codes, which allowed me to dispute charges, was the deciding factor in Medicare's decision to drop all charges. Showing any charges would be paid by Plaintiff rather than Defendant as per Sovereign Immunity Statutes may have also played a part in closing the case.

In addition, I filed a letter with O, the agency retained by AARP, to collect $9,644 of their share of the original $55,562 owed to BCRC. Based on the attached CMS letter, BCRC has determined that the estate of Elizabeth has zero conditional payments owed to BCRC, and their case has been adjusted accordingly. On this basis, O no longer needs to pursue a recovery of medical benefits paid on behalf of Elizabeth, and your case should be closed. It is requested that O issue a formal notice of closure to me.

It was hard to imagine that three months ago, I was facing a $55,562 charge from BCRC and a $9,644 bill from O. My disputing those charges, and proving my contentions, resulted in removing $65,206 from being a factor in my lawsuit.

My review of all the DX codes billed to Medicare by the medical profession shows that many DX codes have no application to the condition. CMS has never had anyone question their 'conditional payments,' as I have, and I am one of the few to have CMS waive payments without a final lawsuit completion.

Chapter 36
Mediation Preparation

On 2 August, my attorney and I discussed tomorrow's mediation. He informed me that he could not find an expert medical witness to defend our position based on HPCC's records. The expert uses HPCC's medical records, which we say are incomplete and lack medical tests justifying their reason for leaving the embedded catheter, which we claim contributed to her death. He stated that without an expert witness, there is no chance of our proceeding with a wrongful death case. I requested that the expert doctor send me the medical records he is using to give his opinion.

The expert bases his opinion on one sentence in the 29 July hospital report: 'patient has failed voiding tests in the past.' This statement comes from HPCC's records sent to the hospital and appears to be a cover-your-ass statement to explain their need for a catheter. After seeing what the doctor used for his opinion, I sent the following e-mail to my attorney.

The expert bases his opinion on the statement, "Pt has failed voiding trials in the past." This statement was made on 1 August, 76 days after the catheter was embedded on 18 May 2017. Records will show that the catheter was implanted without supporting evidence that the resident failed a bladder scan. My review of hundreds of documents shows no notation of the resident failing a voiding the test.

The statement "It has failed voiding trials in the past" is based on information furnished to the hospital by HPCC because there is no record of the hospital performing voiding tests. I repeat once again. The only voiding trials conducted by HPCC show no need for a catheter. The expert is basing his opinion on erroneous information documented to be inaccurate. If this is the only statement on which the expert bases his argument, he still needs to do his homework to determine the basis of those failed voiding trials.

As for the leave the catheter in language, she came into the hospital with an embedded catheter, and Dr. B had only the word of HPCC. The expert needs to read the report from Dr. B, where he questions the need for a catheter and his plan for catheter removal. I suggest you send the completed Mediation Summary showing him the whole story and telling him to expand his investigation beyond the hospital statement on which he is basing his opinion.

It appears vital to find an expert witness agreeing with our position that she did not need the catheter. He must be prepared to counter the defendant's two expert witnesses, who say the catheter was justified. Our case is based on no bladder scanning trials justifying the catheter, so we must find a physician to agree with our contention. The estimated cost of seeing a doctor agreeing with our position was between $3,000 and $5,000. Finding a doctor to contradict another doctor at this late-game stage is nonexistent.

The deep pockets defense can easily find two expert witnesses who will testify that the catheter was justified. In addition to the two experts HPCC can use, they can also use the finding of K, the Medicare Quality of Care vendor I filed my Medicare complaint. As previously described, despite my documented summary that HPCC violated Medicare mandates on using an embedded catheter, K ruled that HPCC followed standard medical practice.

I am now prepared to lower my expectations of any appreciable settlement offer. My attorney told me to prepare talking points detailing our case for presentation to the mediator, but I got carried away with my detail, and the talking points became four pages. Much of what follows has been stated previously in the story, but it would be the first time the mediator would hear it. My talking points are the most detailed description of our case.

HPCC is a Medicare facility that receives millions of dollars in Medicare reimbursement and runs under Medicare's quality of care directives. I want to quote Medicare order CMS 20068. Ensure a resident who enters the facility without an indwelling catheter is not catheterized unless the resident's condition demonstrates that catheterization was necessary.

HPCC knowingly violated that directive by embedding a Foley catheter without a voiding test to determine whether the resident had urine retention. With no testing to determine the necessity of catheterization, the catheter was embedded for the convenience of HPCC to reduce the work on the understaffed and overwork aides.

The second directive on CMS 20068 states. Ensure a resident who enters the facility with an indwelling catheter or subsequently receives one is assessed for removal of the catheter as soon as possible unless the resident's clinical condition demonstrates that catheterization is necessary. The catheter, embedded on 18 May, was still implanted on 29 July, 72 days, when the resident was sent to the hospital in a non-responsive state.

In my review of 184 pages of records from HPCC, there is no mention of the resident failing a voiding test which would be the only reason for leaving the catheter embedded. In fact, on 6/4/17, the nurse's notes state, "bladder scan with no urine in the bladder." During her stay at HPCC, her urologist recommended removing the catheter. His records show no medical evidence that she needed a catheter, and he believes HPCC embedded it for the convenience of the nursing home staff.

Despite having a Foley embedded, he thought her need to urinate neurologic and psychiatric, a belief echoed by the urologist at HPCC, who also stated her opinion on the need to pee, which was the basis for the catheter, was not physical but psychiatric. Two doctors, one a urologist, questioned the need for a chronic catheter and recommended removal in the hospital.

The third directive states that a resident receives appropriate treatment services to prevent urinary tract infections to the extent possible. My wife had a UTI on 26 May and still had it when hospitalized on 29 July. She was treated with various drugs during that period, resulting in the facility declaring that the UTI was drug-resistant.

When she arrived at the hospital, the doctor found the catheter dirty and thought this might cause her UTI. The first evidence is that the embedded catheter may have contributed to her frequent UTIs. Her new facility agreed with her urologist that the catheter was unnecessary, removed it, and successfully treated her UTI.

My final HPCC comment on the risk associated with catheterization. HPCC's Patient Care Plan states that: Problem started on 5/18/17—alteration in urinary elimination and risk for infection r/t indwelling catheter. HPCC knew the risks associated with an embedded catheter—residents' rights under Chapter 400.022 of the Florida Statutes section state.

"Has the right to be adequately informed of their medical condition and proposed treatment, unless the resident is determined to be unable to provide informed consent under Florida law. The right to be fully informed of any nonemergency changes in care or treatment that may affect the resident's well-being. The right to participate in planning medical treatment, including the right to refuse medication and treatment, unless otherwise indicated by the resident's physicians, and to know the consequences of such actions."

My wife was a registered nurse with 40 years of nursing experience, including 15 years of experience in nursing facilities, and thus knew the ramifications of using an indwelling catheter. With that knowledge, there is no way she would have consented to embed a catheter unless medical evidence, such as a bladder scan, showed the treatment was necessary. She never had the opportunity to consent to her treatment. Thus, HP was in direct violation of Chapter 400.022.

Any breach of the residence in this section is grounds for action by the agency under 400.102. Section 400.102 States grounds for action by the agency against the licensee for: "An intentional or negligent act materially affecting the health or safety of residents of the facility."

Medscape states: "Using a Foley catheter for a prolonged period is strongly discouraged. Indwelling urethral catheters are a significant cause of UTIs, and not being treated may lead to urosepsis and death. The death rate of nursing home residents with urethral catheters is three times higher than for residents without."

The Omnibus Budget Reconciliation Act (OBRA), also known as the Nursing Home Reform Act of 1987, is the act that has dramatically improved the quality of care in nursing homes. One of the improvements was reducing the inappropriate use of indwelling catheters. Nursing homes must comply with the federal requirement for nursing homes to participate in Medicare and Medicaid programs.

The failure of a nursing home to comply with the OBRA quality of care mandates in caring for a resident is a failure to exercise the degree of reasonable care and skill they should expect. Such consideration includes only using urinary catheters when proper, as outlined in the regulations, to prevent adverse consequences related to such use. HPCC has violated Medicare and the mandates concerning the use of catheters spelled out in OBRA.

Medical Patient states, "Too many unnecessary catheters are done, and some recipients have died from complications caused by urinary catheters." Foley catheters are an improper treatment for incontinence, my wife's condition. Every patient should be informed about the risks of urinary catheters and offered alternative and less invasive procedures.

For example, a bladder scan can easily measure bladder volume. My wife had a catheter embedded immediately upon arrival at HPCC without being informed of the risks of urinary catheters or shown justification, through a bladder scan, for implanting a catheter.

The article states: "It is quite common for patients to get UTIs from catheters, and some infections can be deadly. A nursing home-acquired UTI is often not a simple infection to treat because the bacteria are more likely to be drug-resistant," as determined by HPCC's doctors.

Health Line states: "A catheter-associated CAUTI is one of the most common infections a person can counter; bacteria or fungi may enter your urinary tract via the catheter, and they can multiply and cause an infection. Catheters should not be left longer than needed, as longer use is associated with a higher risk of infection. Prompt treatment of a CAUTI is essential since an untreated UTI can lead to a more serious kidney infection."

I could quote other health organizations such as *CDC* and *Mayo Clinic*. Still, I have pointed out that embedding a catheter is not a recognized standard medical procedure because of the present and future medical ramifications. After reviewing the detailed facts, I find it incomprehensible how a urologist could make a diagnosis justifying an indefinite-duration embedded catheter. Two years after leaving HPCC, my wife suffered 25 UTIs, 12 of which required hospitalization to cure.

Women in their lifetime will experience the pain of a UTI only 2 to 3 times. With each UTI, her kidney function deteriorated to the point where her kidneys finally failed. I sat with her in hospice for two weeks, where she kept asking, "When can I go home" and: "God, please make me better."

The catheter embedding, in violation of Medicare and OBRA guidelines on the restricted use of an embedded catheter, and the poor management thereof were contributing factors to the death of my wife. Knowing a catheter is one of the significant sources of UTIs, HPCC continued to treat a drug-resistant UTI while leaving the catheter embedded. Using my WebMD, I know to remove the catheter if you cannot cure a UTI with a catheter implanted.

Now I would like to address the dehydration issue. In August 2017, I informed the nursing superintendent that my wife was dehydrated. I supported my findings by showing elevated BUN lab readings, BUN being one of the medical indications of dehydration, and a torque test. Eventually, the staff agreed that my wife needed to be rehydrated intravenously and would start the procedure that night.

Not finding my wife on an IV the following day, I inquired why not. When nurses tried to place an IV, I was told that her veins kept collapsing, and they discontinued trying. They would try to rehydrate her by getting her to drink more. When her condition did not improve, I requested that she be rehydrated in the hospital emergency room. Rather than send her to the hospital, they would find someone to place an IV.

Eventually, they found a male nurse who succeeded in putting in the IV, but it was too late. This description of events shows that HPCC staff had inadequate training in installing an IV. On 29 August, I received a call from HPCC informing me that my wife was found in a non-responsive state and was waiting for the doctor's orders. My wife is near-death, non-responsive, and the nurses await the doctor's orders. He ordered her to be sent to the ER, where the doctors found her severely dehydrated and started aggressive rehydration. In addition, she had a UTI and pneumonia.

Now let me educate you on the potentially life-threatening complications of dehydration. Kidney failure:

When you get severely dehydrated, your blood volume goes down, and your kidneys may shut down to prevent further water loss in your urine. When kidneys remain shut down for too long, they could be permanently damaged. It is unknown how long the plaintiff was non-responsive before being rushed to the hospital, but it was hours. The plaintiff's kidneys shutdown could have damaged her kidneys and contributed to her death from kidney failure.

Brain Injury:

Rapid loss of blood volume and low blood pressure may damage your brain. One reason for HPCC's discharge to the hospital was low blood pressure. My wife did experience memory loss after being aggressively rehydrated by the emergency doctors. I could refer to pages and pages of documentation showing the harm caused by the continued use of a catheter and the severe damage dehydration can cause. Still, I think I have covered the subjects thoroughly. My attorney thought it was an excellent presentation but too long, and he will elect to give a shorter case summary to the mediator.

Mediation is scheduled for three hours, with the mediator being paid an estimated $300 to $600 per hour with a three-hour minimum. I agreed that my talking points would be too time-consuming and would let my attorney make the opening statement. They are the most concise description of our case, but the mediator is there only to get a brief background on the subject and not to decide the case's merits.

Much of my talking points have been made previously, but this is my last opportunity to summarize them. As detailed as my summary is, I would not be allowed to present it at trial because only a medical doctor can state what I have just described.

Let me digress here. This case started as a medical malpractice lawsuit, and we had HPCC nurses' notes and medical reports justifying our malpractice allegations. Medical Malpractice refers to a healthcare facility deviating from the expected standard of care, whether by negligence or intentional act, and that deviation causes injury to the resident. All care facilities are expected to adhere to this standard of care.

Deviating from this standard or neglecting to perform to that standard of care usually results in a medical malpractice claim. A claim can be for either Medical Negligence, which does not require the patient to be injured or Medical Malpractice, where the patient suffered harm. Our claim met the requirements of being a Medical Malpractice claim. We had an excellent case and would have gotten a reasonable settlement in mediation.

However, when Beth died, everything changed. The issue now goes from a Medical Malpractice claim to a Wrongful Death claim, a tough lawsuit to win. In the malpractice case, we had all the evidence needed to present our case, but the evidence required changes in a wrongful death case.

The Florida Statutes 766.102 states: In any action for recovery of damages based on the death of any person in which it is alleged such death resulted from the negligence of a health care provider, *the claimant shall have the burden of proving by the greater weight of evidence* the alleged actions of the health care provider represented a breach of prevailing professional standard of care for that health care provider.

The general professional standard of care for a given health care provider shall be that level of care that, considering all relevant surrounding circumstances, is recognized as acceptable and appropriate. Suppose the injury is claimed to have resulted from the negligent affirmative medical intervention of the health care provider. In that case, the claimant must prove a breach of the prevailing professional standard of care.

In any claim brought according to alleging a violation of a resident's rights or negligence causing the death of a resident, *the claimant shall have the burden of proving, by a preponderance of the evidence,* that: The defendant owed a duty to the resident, the defendant breached that duty, the breach is a legal cause of death, and the resident's death was a result of the violation. *If the plaintiff does not meet the burden on any of the elements of negligence, the plaintiff will not recover any damages.*

Here, I refer to my filing of the quality-of-care complaint with K and why I was adamant about showing that their conclusions were wrong. K's decision that the actions of HPCC were within the prevailing professional standard of care can be referred to by HPCC to show that their efforts were not contributing to the plaintiff's death. *We now have the burden of proving that the medical malpractice evidence we presented was the direct cause of Beth's death.*

A burden of proof we did not have and could only obtain by retaining doctors, at an estimated $3,000 to $5,000 retainer fee, to agree with our allegations. The task of getting a doctor to testify against another doctor is dreaming. We now basically go into mediation with no case.

Both attorneys knew these facts when this became a wrongful death case in July 2019 but continued to file meaningless court documents over the next two years. The case, upon her death, could have been settled for a nominal amount and years of court procedures eliminated.

As mentioned previously, the defendant had no incentive to settle the case, being on a retainer. The delaying tactics of the defense accomplished their goal of running up the expenses of the plaintiff responding to each delay and thus discouraging any attorney from litigating a Florida Sovereign Immunity lawsuit, leaving many valid medical malpractice cases un-litigated.

Chapter 37
Mediation

On 3 August, I entered ZOOM to join my attorney and the mediator for the scheduled mediation. The mediator's primary purpose is to help outline the issue and facilitate communication so the parties can hopefully agree to a mutually beneficial settlement. The mediator is not there to give legal advice. He wanted a case summary without the defendant attending to update him.

Having agreed that my prepared presentation was too long, my attorney gave a shorter version of the case. He advised us that he was not there to decide the validity of our claims but only to seek an agreed-upon settlement. His primary purpose was to take settlement offers and return with counteroffers from the plaintiff and defendant. Defense counsel then came on screen and presented their case. There are confidentiality rules governing what mediation communications can be disclosed, but the nature of the defendant's case was already known to us, so it is not confidential.

They stated that the plaintiff did not show the lasting effects of the catheter and dehydration issues. They referred to K's report that decided HPCC's procedures met the medical standard of care, and HPCC's two medical experts would support that contention. Their final exhibit was the death certificate which determined Beth died from Alzheimer's.

One known disadvantage of mediation is that it infrequently reveals the complete truth of an issue. As suspected, not being able to counter their evidence, and with the burden of proof being upon the plaintiff to show HPCC's medical malpractice was the cause of the plaintiff's death, we had a weak case.

Referring to the confidential clause, let us assume all figures used here are hypothetical. Naturally, the plaintiff will ask for the $200,000 cap on damages, and the defense will either not accept the amount or counter it. For the next three hours, the high-priced mediator's job is to take the demands of the plaintiff and the defendant counter between the parties.

There were numerous proposals and counters in that three hours, but let us make the hypothetical assumption that the plaintiff's final demands had dropped to $20,000, and the defendant's last offer was $10,000.

Let me here express my dissatisfaction with my attorney's negations. He did not set a bottom dollar value from which we would negotiate.

Assume that figure would be $50,000, giving us greater leeway in negotiating against the defendant's $10,000 offer, with the possible compromise being $30,000, the midpoint. By my attorney dropping our demands quickly to $20,000, he showed he had a weak case, and rather than negotiating, he was capitulating to the defendant. Our negotiating for a compromise midpoint settlement was now limited to $15,000.

Settlement amounts are confidential, but the reader knows the hypothetical settlement was between $10,000 and $20,000. We should have ended mediation and gone home when negotiations reached these figures. Still, we had already committed to a hypothetical $20,000 settlement, a great deal for the defendant, so there is no chance we would have been successful in ending mediation without a compromise. The mediator wanted to settle this case to add to his resume and would have discouraged our leaving.

One of the most significant disadvantages of mediation is that it can be challenging to ensure the settlement is fair to both parties. Suppose one party has access to more resources, like the hospital's medical experts and the long form of the death certificate.

In that case, they may get the other party to agree to a settlement that isn't in their best interest. In mediation, there is no discovery process like in a court, and there is no formal method for the plaintiff to acquire the plaintiff's information during mediation.

Court mandate mediation favors the defendant, not the plaintiff, especially in a sovereign immunity case. The defendant knows their maximum exposure is $200,000, and their attorney's sole objective is to reduce that number as low as the plaintiff will accept.

The plaintiff has no bargaining position knowing the purpose of mediation is to reach an acceptable settlement below the $200,000 cap on damages. The defendant, knowing this, never made a settlement offer in the three years of litigation.

Chapter 38
Post Mediation

With both attorneys knowing that as soon as Beth died, the burden of proof now fell upon the plaintiff to prove the malpractice caused the plaintiff's death; the defendant could have offered the same settlement two years ago. Instead, the attorneys produced Complaints, Amended Complaints, Motions to Dismiss, and numerous other legal documents that added legal fees for the defendant's counsel and hours of non-compensated work for the plaintiff.

Like the military, I decided to do an after-action review of the defendant's statements absolving them of any fault in Beth's death. My attorney took the wrong approach when seeking a medical expert who would refute the defendant's Foley catheter use.

He should have agreed with the defendant's placing the catheter, provided she medically needed it. The key phrase is 'proving she medically needed it.' None of HPCC's records show that bladder scans were conducted, showing justification for embedding a catheter. By the defendant's inability to establish the necessity for the catheter, we would have neutralized their medical expert.

As for their reliance on K's report, HPCC's actions met all standard medical practices. By their Medicare directives, we could counter that K relies only on information provided to them by the provider and does not rely on complaint documentation that shows data provided by HPCC was incorrect. Two examples would be.

HPCC's statement Beth transferred from the hospital with a catheter when hospital documentation showed the removal of the catheter. The second example was her being transported to the emergency room in a non-responsive condition, and HPCC's records show her being sent because of low blood pressure.

Their reference to the death certificate shows the cause of death is Alzheimer's. People don't die of Alzheimer's, but that is probably the definitive cause of death listed on a death certificate for patients dying in hospice. Beth was moved from an LMHS hospital to hospice with a diagnosis by LMHS doctors that she was in terminal fifth-stage kidney failure.

We had slam-dunk documentation to win a medical malpractice lawsuit, but it still does not meet the burden of proof needed to show that HPCC's malpractice was the cause of her death. A bar we could not jump over. HPCC was guilty of medical malpractice, but only an autopsy would allow us to show them to be.

By issuing a Freedom of Information Request to the hospital, I could get a summary of the fee paid to the outside counsel retained to prosecute the lawsuit. He was paid $26,894 for his services plus $579 in legal fees. My counsel, who spent the same three years preparing meaningless court documents to answer the defendant's delays, earned $2,500.

Is it obvious why attorneys are reluctant to take sovereign immunity lawsuits? My costs taken out of the settlement were the $2,500 contingency fee, $5,425 in legal fees, much less than I expected, $2,800 in probate expenses, and $150 for postage and document purchases for a total of $10,875.

Picture this. The defense attorney made more money defending HPCC, the medical malpractice defendant than the plaintiff, whose wife died due to HPCC's medical malpractice, made from the LMHS settlement. I am sure LMHS would not like the public to know this information.

Money is not the only reason aggrieved parties file lawsuits. In my case, it was to get HPCC to admit to settling a wrongful death lawsuit. I realize a monetary settlement will be written off as a cost of doing business, but I was hoping to publicize that LMHS had settled a wrongful death lawsuit.

When a medical facility settles a wrongful death lawsuit, they are to report it to Florida's Agency for Health Care Administration to be placed on its record and be available to anyone searching the history of that facility's lawsuits. However, this case was dismissed with precedence and need not be reported to AHCA.

My other attempt to publicize was through the newspaper. Surprisingly I was not bound by a non-disclosure agreement.

The settlement agreement stated, "The undersigned shall refrain from making any written or oral statement known to be disparaging or negative concerning LMHS's actions concerning the alleged medical negligence and alleged violation of resident rights, except the undersigned may provide truthful information in response to a valid subpoena or other legal processes."

Interpreting this statement literary, I decided to once again seek to inform, through an op-ed, the public of LMHS's wrongful death settlement and to educate them on Florida's Sovereign Immunity Statutes. Except for the first paragraph, the op-ed was the same as previously submitted.

The opening line now reads, "After delaying litigation for three and a half years, LMHS, on 3 August, in court-ordered mediation, agreed to a settlement in a wrongful death lawsuit filed against the defendant HPCC. The lawsuit fell under Florida's Sovereign Immunity Statutes, statutes detailed as follows:" Here, staying within the 600-word limit, I explained the statute. Op-ed rejected.

You are reading my final attempt to inform you of the wrongful death settlement and educate you on the statutes. I realize that writing a book may not fall under the guidelines detailed in the hospital release, and I could be subject to legal action. If so, there is a good chance any lawsuit would outlive me.

I also contacted the Medical Director at K, with whom I had my conference, to see if they would like to know the final results of the lawsuit. They informed me they would, and I sent them the same opening paragraph from my op-ed and included the presentation I had prepared for the mediator. I added.

I am sure you wondered why I was adamant about critiquing K's quality of care complaint investigation procedure. Here is why. HPCC is a Medicare facility that knowingly violated Medicare's CMS 20068 mandate on the limited use of catheters but will still collect millions of dollars in Medicare reimbursements yearly. The monetary judgment to settle a wrongful death case will be written off as a cost of doing business. It will not be an incentive for HPCC to change their catheter use without medical justification, especially with K's approval that such a practice met medical standards for future residents.

Your investigation procedures, which accept the records of the charged facility as factual while ignoring the medical documentation submitted by the complainant, are biased toward the accused. Your investigation procedures were not only unfair to me but will be unfair to future complainants. As per your stated investigation methods of only investigating one side of the story based on the accused's medical records, I cannot accept K's investigation decisions as unbiased.

The only punishment that would get HPCC to change their continued use of a catheter without medical justification would be Medicare sanctions. Based on the medical documentation I submitted, these were such sanctions that I expected K to recommend. By not doing so, K condones HPCCs practice of indwelling catheters without bladder scan documentation. K's reply again complimented me on my being so concerned about my wife's medical treatment.

Chapter 39
Brief Case Summary

In July 2019, Beth's two years of pain and suffering ended in hospice, and after three years of trying to prove the king could do no harm, it ended with the king in August 2021 paying a minimum monetary penalty for the two years of Beth's suffering. What did the readers of this odyssey and I learn? We learned that a hospital in Florida, under sovereign immunity, can remove the wrong kidney in surgery, and the most they can be liable for in a lawsuit is $200,000.

We learned these facts from Florida's malpractice laws written not to benefit the kidney patient but to benefit insurance companies, hospitals, and doctors. These laws make it exceedingly difficult to pursue a medical malpractice case and even more challenging to find a law firm willing to take the time and effort to do so, knowing their limited recovery compensation.

Medical malpractice cases are time-consuming and expensive to litigate, so it makes no economic sense for a law firm to pursue a sovereign immunity case. Often the issues are turned down even though the malpractice was egregious and led to someone's death.

The same king can do no harm statute applies to wrongful death. One can die in a botched operation, and the same $200,000 pain and suffering maximum damages still applies. To quote articles researched on the web, I find the following statements prevalent in all of them.

"Because Florida's medical, hospital, and insurance industries are very politically powerful, the law allows such patients to be killed by medical negligence without recourse. The medical, hospital, and insurance industries lobby, donate, and are given what they want in the name of the false battle cry of eliminating frivolous lawsuits and tort reform." Following is a summary of the Wrongful Death Lawsuit saga that commenced in May 2017 and ended in August 2021.

It started with my wife going to the hospital after a May 2017 fall at home, where the doctor misread an x-ray, and the discharge nurse did not perform a proper 'road test'; she sent her home with a broken leg. Arriving home and placing weight on the injured leg, Beth collapsed, necessitating a 911 call for EMS assistance to get her up and into bed.

After a night of excruciating pain and the failure of LMHS to schedule a home health nurse to check on her, EMS returned her to the hospital, where an ultrasound found she had a broken tibia/fibula. Her surgeon later determined that what was a possible tibia fracture had become a fractured, shattered tibia/fibula with an estimated 4-to-5-month recovery period to allow the bones to grow back together naturally.

Beth moved to HPCC for skilled nursing and rehab, where the facility's actions constituted medical malpractice. Upon arrival and directly violating Medicare guidelines on using catheters, HPCC embedded a catheter without any medical justification. We contend that the catheter was implanted not for medical reasons but for the benefit of the aides not having to take Beth to the bathroom or, what would have been the medically approved treatment, change her diaper.

For the next sixty days, while the catheter remained embedded, she suffered persistent urinary tract infections (UTIs), which the doctors found drug-resistant. Medicare states that if a catheter must be medically implanted, it be removed as quickly as possible.

Ignoring these directives, Beth suffered a continuous UTI and an urge to urinate despite the catheter being embedded continuously. The medical profession unanimously agrees that catheters are the most significant source of UTIs; advice HPCC ignored.

She became severely dehydrated during her stay at HPCC, needing IV rehydration. When the nursing staff attempted to place an IV, they could not perform the procedure and decided to rehydrate her by getting her to drink more. My wife returned to the emergency room in a near-death non-responsive condition, where the hospital doctor started aggressive rehydration.

After a four-day hospital stay, HPCC denied her reentry, saying no beds were available. The facility sending Beth to the hospital because of their medical malfeasance states she cannot return. A new rehab, on short notice, was found, and they immediately removed the catheter determining it was not medically necessary.

Determining I had a possible medical malpractice case against the hospital and the nursing home, I started a search for legal representation. Based on the events described above, I expected no problem finding an attorney to take the case, and I was wrong because of 'Florida's Sovereign Immunity Statutes.'

I have detailed FSIS throughout my story, so I will not elaborate on them in summary. I also documented my attempt to educate Florida citizens, especially those in the county using the LMHS, the most extensive health system in southwest Florida, about their being affected by the statutes if they use hospitals, nursing homes, or doctors associated with LMHS.

This attempt to educate consisted of three 600-word op-eds and three Letters to the Editor submitted to the local newspaper, all of which the paper declined to publish. Their refusal to print probably made LMHS happy since their failure to publish kept the county's citizens ignorant of FSIS.

After weeks of searching for legal representation, even being turned down by the firm that advertises as being 'for the people,' as soon as they realized it was an FSIS case without giving me my free consultation, I located a firm in Tampa willing to take the case. I doubt they knew it was an FSIS case, as evidenced by having three different attorneys before they settled the matter.

After the case was assigned a case number for the next three-plus years, the attorneys submitted ninety-nine (99) documents consisting of 396 pages of legalese to the court consisting of Complaints, Amended Complaints, Second Complaints, Third Complaints, each followed by the defendant's Motion to Dismiss.

Attorneys could have eliminated documentation since both knew the case would never see the inside of a courtroom. However, as mentioned, the defense attorney is on a retainer from LMHS; a quick settlement of the case would have substantially reduced his legal fees.

The death of the plaintiff, my wife, in July 2019 ended the medical malpractice lawsuit, and it became a wrongful death lawsuit. Her death changed the momentum of the suit from the plaintiff to the defendant. There is something wrong with the legal system when the death of a plaintiff ends up favoring the defendant—so much for equal justice under the law.

Knowing a monetary settlement made by HPCC would just be considered a cost of doing business; I filed a formal 'Quality of Care Complaint' with the agency retained by Medicare to investigate such complaints. By presenting my malpractice complaints to the agency, I sought to get them to agree that the quality of care did not meet Medicare standards.

The agency would then recommend Medicare sanctions, a penalty far more devastating to HPCC than a monetary settlement. I was disappointed again when the agency determined that the actions of HPCC met all the standards of acceptable medical care.

Per their investigative process, their findings state, "Only the reports submitted by HPCC will be accepted as fact in determining the care given, and it is not up to the agency to determine whether those reports are accurate." It also states that despite my documentation of HPCC's misconduct, "the documentation by the complaint will not have a bearing on the vendors' determination whether they followed proper medical practices." Another strike against the plaintiff.

Next was the hard-to-believe scenario of Medicare and AARP Insurance informing me that I would have to pay $55,000 and $9,000 of medical payments made on a conditional basis to LMHS out of any settlement I may get from LMHS.

Consider this, amounts of money paid by Medicare and AARP to LMHS were to be reimbursed to Medicare and AARP by me. Repeat, not to be repaid by LMHS, the recipient of the funding, but by me. Please consider this scenario; I could win a medical malpractice settlement from LMHS and owe Medicare and AARP tens of thousands of dollars. Is there something wrong with this picture?

Finally, after years of unnecessary claims, motions, depositions, and other documents making up the ninety-nine documents submitted to the court, the case ends in court-mandated mediation. Mediation, which benefits the defendant at the plaintiff's expense, is overseen by a mediator making an estimated $1,800 to take the offers of the plaintiff and the defendant from room to room.

With LMHS, the deep pockets defendant, having expert witnesses, reports from the Medicare investigating agency, and a long form of the death certificate, and the plaintiff's need for a preponderance of evidence showing the medical malpractice being the cause of the plaintiff's death, the defendant can squash the plaintiff. This mediation process conducted in August of 2021 could have been completed in July 2019 upon the death of my wife when the attorneys knew the same facts presented here. It is a long trip through the halls of justice.

Having experienced seeing the workings of five different assisted living and nursing homes, I can comment on my experience. First are my comments on the state inspections of nursing homes. It is OK to have a detailed review procedure, but what infractions occur between inspections, for instance, using a resident catheter?

In that case, the checks accomplish very little unless the deficiencies are evident during the inspection. I was the one who discovered the implanting of a non-medically needed catheter and not by any state inspection. How many resident representatives are capable of making such a discovery?

I must also emphasize the need for long-term nursing care insurance. Assisted living and long-term care nursing homes are costly, and both profit and not-for-profit nursing homes have the same problem, staffing. The more expensive the facility usually results in better care, mainly because they can pay their aides more, an essential aspect of nursing care, and retain staff.

The non-profits rely on aides from Porto Rice, Haiti, Honduras, or other Caribbean countries. Language problems sometimes make it difficult for the resident and aide to communicate. Most of the aides cared and provided good care, but in many cases, aide turnover prevented an aide and resident from getting to know each other. I must admit that the theft of my wife's diamond wedding ring did not enhance my endorsement of some of the aides.

One of the essential elements in choosing nursing home care is the food and the dining facility. You may think this to be low on the evaluation scale, but having decent food is one of the only times a resident can relax and at least sit with other people in a relaxing setting. The setting and the process of feeding residents differed in each facility.

In one, the residents choose two meals and sit in a well-lighted colorful dining room with three other residents. The meals are brought from the kitchen and served on brightly colored tablecloths. A bright dining room allows the residents to sit and chat for a while before returning to their rooms. This facility was the best of the five and the most expensive for-profit facility. Food was brought into a non-descript dining room in other facilities and served from a serving cart to the residents.

In some facilities, the food was unappetizing and lukewarm, served between 11:00 and 1:00 for lunch and 5:00 to 7:00 for dinner, and the ice cream in a paper cup melted. In these facilities, the residents ate what they could and immediately returned to their room or elected not to go to the dining room and take meals.

Finally, I cannot speak highly enough about hospice care. The care and service provided to Beth in the final weeks of her life exceeded my expectations. She could not have passed away in a more serene setting, and I continue to praise the care and comfort she received in her final days. In appreciation for that care, 25% of any book royalties I may receive will be donated to hospice.

Yes, I got a damage award against HPCC, but it is hard to consider any settlement as an award. I see it more as punishment to the LMHS, but even then, how can you punish a firm with monetary damages that amount to petty cash to the hospital? It is impossible to value an individual's pain and suffering unless you can experience it yourself.

How can an independent legislature determine that medical misconduct resulting in losing a loved one is only worth $200,000? If the case described here were against a hospital or nursing home not covered by sovereign immunity, there would be no cap on damages, and it would be up to a jury to determent the value for the pain and suffering and the loss of a loved one. These caps are a prime example of why law firms are reluctant to enter lawsuits against the king, who can do no wrong.

Many claims are refused because it makes no economic sense for an attorney to pursue an expensive FSIS medical malpractice case, even though the malpractice was egregious and led to someone's death. The laws should be consistent across the board and treat a sovereign immunity case no different from a lawsuit against a defendant not protected by that statute; today, the law is not fair.

The law should be consistent, and everyone deserves a fair day in court. Under sovereign immunity, constancy is impossible and will only change if the Florida legislature recognizes that aggrieved plaintiffs in a sovereign immunity case deserve a statute change.

While authoring this story, I read about a South Carolina wrongful death lawsuit where the jury awarded the plaintiff $4.3 million. In that case, the law firm may have spent about the same amount of time as my attorney did on my case.

It becomes evident why attorneys are reluctant to take sovereign immunity cases and why sovereign immunity entities choose to settle claims in mediation rather than take their chances on a jury trial. Even the pit bull in St. Louis got $750,000 for his wrongful death lawsuit.

I have documented, without any doubt, that HPCC committed medical malpractice by embedding a catheter and leaving it embedded for a period far exceeding Medicare guidelines.

Such malpractice was a contributing factor to my wife's death. The sad part of this lawsuit is that, although I have documented HPCC's misconduct, the suit will do nothing to ensure the same misconduct is not practiced on other residents.

Chapter 40
Conclusion

It has been four years since Beth fell, and my journey through the halls of justice-seeking redress for medical malpractice has ended. A journey that could have ended in March 2019 while Beth was still alive, and she could have seen we extracted some justice for all her pain and suffering. Was the trip worth it for me? Moneywise, no, but that was not the sole purpose of the suit. People typically begin lawsuits for money, but more than money is at stake.

The plaintiffs feel aggrieved; the defendants are affronted. The plaintiff wants the damage settlement to incentivize the offending party to correct their wrongdoing and ensure it does not happen again to another injured party. In this case, does a small monetary settlement accomplish that goal for a nursing home receiving millions of dollars in Medicare reimbursement annually, or will the payment be a rounding error on the nursing home's balance sheet?

The Florida legislature accomplished what the medical profession wanted by adopting the Sovereign Immunity Statutes. It established that regardless of the fault of the medical practitioner, you, the recipient of the malpractice, will only be entitled to a $200,000 damage settlement, irrespective of whether that malpractice costs the plaintiff figures far more than the $200,000 for medical fees to treat the consequences of that malpractice. For sovereign immunity agencies like LMHS, the settlement amount is considered a cost of doing business.

As for getting the maximum settlement, fat chance, with court-ordered mediation, the defendant's attorney's job is to get that figure as low as possible and the plaintiff to agree to a figure much lower than the offense dictated. Usually, at this point, the defense's delays have dragged the case well beyond where it should have ended, thus running the plaintiff's expenses up with each pause. In this case, the defendant had deep pockets and could pay outside counsel $27,473 in retainer fees and costs.

The plaintiff's attorney has to deal with all these delays while making $2,500 for three and half years of work. A law firm cannot stay in business prosecuting a case like this, and it is a prime example of why so few attorneys are willing to take a Florida sovereign immunity lawsuit. Making it much worse, the defendant is a public agency, and thus they are spending my $27,473 to litigate against me.

As an aside, LMHS ended its budget year in September 2021, taking in about $160 million more than it spent. Much of this money was from Medicare and Medicaid programs reimbursement. The same Medicare mandates they ignored when treating my wife. You can see where in *this David versus Goliath story how Goliath was able to purchase bigger stones.*

The defendant knew the case would never proceed to trial because they would not want the publicity. I tried to nullify this by sending op-eds to the newspaper exposing the hospital's settlement of a wrongful death suit and educating the public on Florida's Sovereign Immunity Statutes. I tried to do the same with a Letter to the Editor, also to no avail.

I tried to make the defendant report the wrongful death suit settlement to the state agency by issuing a Freedom of Information Request for a copy of the documents submitted to the agency. However, since the case was dismissed with prejudice, it did not have to be reported to the agency.

Did I have the sharpest legal firm on my side? Who knows, since I had three different attorneys from the same firm? As mentioned, big firms will not take a sovereign immunity case because of the tactics the defense can use during the legal process. My third attorney did an excellent job prosecuting the case, but going up against a hospital is like the pre-mentioned David vs. Goliath story, with Goliath having the bigger stones this time.

I would have loved to have taken this case to court, especially with women on the jury. Just describing the number of UTIs my wife suffered would have made the case, I believe, a slam dunk. I knew there was never a chance the defendant would ever let this case proceed to a jury trial, so all my and my attorney's preparation was for naught.

Did the plaintiff prove, without any doubt, that HPCC's medical malfeasance was the contributing cause of Beth's death? I believe we documented with medical records and statements made in the HPCC's nurse's notes.

Did I accomplish my goal of informing the public of the nursing home settling a wrongful death lawsuit? No. Did I achieve my goal of educating the public about Florida's Sovereign Immunity Statutes? No. Did my suing HPCC for their medical malpractice change their use of embedded catheters on future residents? We will never know.

Was it worth it? It was, in a way, because it took up my time while my wife was suffering and kept me busy after her death. I could take this opportunity to expose the county's citizens to Florida's Sovereign Immunity Statutes and the iniquity thereof to the injured parties that may suffer lifelong pain or death. However, as previously mentioned, I even failed in this quest. My wife is still dead after suffering years of pain because of the known negligence of HPCC, and any money I get will never change that.

What did I learn? You will have a challenging time trying to beat the system. They have no problem getting expert witnesses to justify their actions, thus forcing the plaintiff to find witnesses to counter their witnesses. The defendant accomplishes their goal of making it so expensive for the plaintiff to prosecute the case that the plaintiff throws up his hands and says settle.

Based on all the medical documentation needed, we did have the *'smoking gun'* evidence necessary to find the defendant liable for medical malpractice. However, for a wrongful death case, we needed to have the *'bullet'* that exited that gun and prove that bullet caused the plaintiff's death by the preponderance of the evidence.

So much for equal justice under the law.

I did accomplish one goal; I outlived the lawsuit.

Chapter 41
Postscript

On 2 January 2022, the local newspaper posted an article entitled 'Dear Readers: Please Write Us.' The jest of the story was that the paper staff was upset because too many of the Letters to the Editor are about highly controversial state and national politics, not local issues. His plea prompted me to submit the following letter once again.

In the past few months, I have submitted three op-eds, changing the first paragraph each time to skirt possible legal ramifications, and two Letters to the Editor covering the same subject, none printed by the paper. David states he is looking for more local issues. The subject of my op-eds, Florida's Sovereign Immunity Statutes, applies to the whole state but mainly to anyone locally using the LMHS.

I consider myself very knowledgeable on the statutes, having just settled a three-and-a-half-year wrongful death litigation in mediation which, by doing so, prevents the public from knowledge of the defendant's settlement. It would have been a front-page, above-the-fold news story if a jury had awarded the compensation. LMHS is a political subdivision of the state, created by the Florida legislature, and is protected by Florida's Sovereign Immunity Statutes.

The statute is too long to detail in a letter but was covered in my op-eds previously mentioned. 99% of the county population have yet to learn they are subject to the statutes when filing a medical malpractice suit against any LH hospital, nursing home, or doctor, and I am sure LMHS would like to keep it that way. This letter is not submitted for publication but to get David to recognize that Sovereign Immunity Statutes are a local issue.

This may be my last chance to expose the county's citizens to their being subject to the statutes. The above letter resulted in an e-mail from the recipient telling me he was the letter to the Editor staffer and that my op-eds should be submitted to the op-ed editor. Having already sent my three versions of the op-ed, I decided to try again.

I sent the same op-ed detailed in Chapter 31. As expected, there was no response, nor was the op-ed printed. The op-ed addresses the local issue the newspaper was seeking, but I must assume the hospital system is mightier than that of the public that the newspaper aims to represent. I have failed once again to educate the county's citizens about FSIS.